# 265 POINT

## TAMARA M. JACKSON

ISBN: 149446537X
ISBN-13: 978-1494465377

# DEDICATION

This book is dedicated to my "angels" - Mary Lenora Bell, Carrie Johnson, and Diane Revis. To this day, memories of you remain a source of immeasurable strength. Rest in peace.

# PREFACE

I decided to write this book after years of being asked how I lost the weight and managed to keep it off. Each time I was asked, I struggled to communicate all of the things I learned during the course of my 12+ year journey into a series of short, but insightful sentences. This book gives me the space and the time to finally share my story and hopefully inspire women around the world to finally and forever shed the weight - mentally, emotionally, and physically.

In 265 Point, I talk about the point – that moment when you've had enough. No more delays, no more denials, no more excuses. That point where you are really and truly ready for change. You're ready to stop "sleepwalking" and you're done with quick fixes. It's no longer about dieting, but about making sustainable changes. It's about designing a new life. It's that point when the pain of your current circumstances – the anger, the depression, the low self-esteem, the unfulfilled dreams – outweigh the pain of charting a new course. The point is a place where you resolve to forge ahead and never look back.

This book was written for those that have reached the point and those that are not yet there. If you have already reached your point of no return, I want to help you stay "on point." If you have yet to arrive, I want to get you there. If you are somewhere in between –

having reached the point but later suffered a relapse – this book is for you too. I've been where you are and I can help.

265 Point is part biography, part education, part inspiration and motivation. I've done my best to assemble the elements necessary for you to succeed.

You will learn:

- Why traditional dieting doesn't work.
- How to find and keep your motivation.
- The real reason you keep sabotaging yourself.
- How to handle unsupportive family and friends.
- Practical ways to silence "the voice" that seeks to protect you but really sets you up for failure, every time.
- Simple steps you can take now to salvage your future through the power of choice.
- How to stop short-circuiting your progress with unrealistic expectations and unhealthy comparisons.
- Easy ways to identify better food choices when eating out.
- Why exercise alone is not enough to get and keep you fit and fly.
- How to reprogram your brain to see the best in you rather than the worst in you.
- What really drives your sense of dignity and your self-confidence (hint: it's not what you think).
- How to enjoy your favorite foods without interfering with your goals using my 80/20 plan.

Writing this book was a bit of a purging process. It forced me to think through and acknowledge some things on paper that I never truly owned up to. It's funny how God works. Often His instruction has a dual purpose. I thought that writing the book was solely to help others. It turns out that it was to help me too. It helped me to get closure on some things and move on. 265 Point was a part of the healing process for me; I hope it will be for you too.

Throughout 265 Point you will see references to various articles, books, and studies. I thought it important to provide sound data, research and insight into the health and fitness methodologies so that you can cut through the crap and walk away inspired and informed. You'll also get a glimpse into the personal experiences that have shaped my outlook on healthy living. I am on a journey; I haven't figured it all out. Still, I'm thankful for how far I've come and optimistic about the days ahead.

I encourage you to take your time as you read this book. Consider it a marathon, not a sprint. Read the "Reflection Points" at the end of each chapter and jot down your thoughts in a journal before moving on. Taking the time to do this is what will make this time different from all the rest.

No matter how many times you've failed, you can do it. It IS possible. You just have to believe the right things. Don't believe the lie. You can change and your change begins now.

*There are no limits, except for those we impose upon ourselves.*
*~Dr. Walter Bishop*

# TABLE OF CONTENTS

Dedication     iii

Preface     iv

Introduction     xi

PART 1 – Emotional Rollercoaster

Before finding success with weight loss, I experienced a range of feelings and emotions. Can you identify with where I was?

**Chapter 1 - Denial: A Great Place**     1
*It's so much easier to deny than to confront.*

**Chapter 2 – Temporary Fix**     13
*A weight loss competition at work inspires change…temporarily.*

**Chapter 3 – Me? No, Not Me. Me?**     18
*I had no idea the situation was that bad. Now what?*

**Chapter 4 – Great Ideas But Why Am I Confused?**     24
*There was so much information, how do I know what works?*

**Chapter 5 – This Can't Be Real**     31
*An answer appears, but was it for real?*

**Chapter 6 – C'mon, It's A White Lie**     36
*It was supposed to be teambuilding, but instead of feeling included, I felt excluded.*

**Chapter 7 – This Is Just Wrong!**     43
*All this work and nothing! Bring on the pity party.*

## PART 2: Oxygen

In the midst of pursuing a happier, healthier life, I encountered many things I didn't expect. It was a challenging, yet incredibility empowering learning experience that I'll never forget.

**Chapter 8 – I Found Answers** 49
*A fresh perspective causes me to look at my situation differently.*

**Chapter 9 – I Think I'm Happy** 59
*I feel empowered. Finally, no more guess work!*

**Chapter 10 – I Knew It Wouldn't Be Easy** 71
*Weight loss was made simple (but not easy). But could I do it?*

**Chapter 11 – The Unexpected** 93
*Someone noticed. It was exciting and eerie at the same time.*

**Chapter 12 – The Intervention** 99
*Help comes from an unexpected place.*

**Chapter 13 – So This Is What Success Feels Like** 107
*My clothes were falling off – yeah!! But I didn't realize this would come along with it.*

**Chapter 14 – Fearing Fear** 112
*Can I really keep this up with the holiday season right around the corner?*

**Chapter 15 – 80/20** 120
*Out of my anxiety, the 80/20 rule was born.*

## PART 3: Looking Good

Finally I was free! The weight was gone! I felt and looked like a new person – inside and out.

**Chapter 16 – I Like the Mirror**                          127

*For the first time in years, I was pleased with how I looked.*

**Chapter 17 – Something New – Pride**                       133

*I believed in myself again. I could change!*

**Chapter 18 – Inhaling Power**                              139

*They say knowledge is power and I couldn't agree more.*

**Chapter 19 – Love This Thing Called "Confidence"**         149

*The healthier me interviewed and dated with a new confidence.*

**Chapter 20 – Gutsy Girl Emerges**                          158

*I found that I enjoyed zip lining and white water rafting – who knew?*

**Chapter 21 – Addicted to Energy**                          165

*I'm feeling lighter and stronger – mentally and physically.*

**Chapter 22 – Mind Relief**                                 171

*My blood pressure was now normal. Finally, I can breathe!*

**Realistic Journey**                                        179

**Appendix/Worksheets**                                      181

# Introduction

Reliving the last 39 years of my life to write this book was trying to say the least. Facing the childhood insecurities, my poor choices in the love department, and my decision to medicate my pain with food, were all tough to resurface and detail. I somehow thought that I had dealt with all of my demons, but it turns out that there were a few lurking in the shadows waiting for the appointed time to be addressed. That time is now.

265 Point has afforded me the opportunity to confront unresolved issues in my past and deal with lingering self-doubt. Some of the issues were relatively easy to sort out; others are still a work in progress. I am still a work in progress.

You see, one does not gain 100+ pounds and lose it without having any scars. I've had the wind knocked out of me more than a time or two. On a few occasions I just laid there on the canvas watching the referee count. Sometimes I honestly wanted to take the TKO. I was exhausted from battle, in pain, disoriented, and less than fully conscious. But each time something rose within me and I got up; I started moving again. There is, however, a difference between getting up and fighting – fighting for your hopes and dreams, for your most important relationships, for your health, and for your life. I had been emaciated by my failures, anxieties, and fears. For 8 years of my life, I existed rather than truly living – and I don't regret any of it.

I don't believe in coincidences. To everything there is a time, a season, and for everything there is a reason. I believe the reason I lived through what I lived through was so that I could share my journey with you, in this book and at this time. It hasn't been easy, but if my story can help one person find value in their life to move forward, then it's been worth recounting every experience and shedding every tear.

# PART I: EMOTIONAL ROLLERCOASTER

"If my life were a song it would probably be titled 'Roller Coaster,'
up and down all the time."
~Scotty McCreery

# Chapter 1 - Denial: A Great Place

It was winter, 2007. My doctor looked at me and said, "You realize you're a disaster waiting to happen, don't you?" If that wasn't bad enough he added, "It's only a matter of time before you end up really sick or worse." Worse?? What's worse? Death! He meant death. I was 33 years old, what is wrong with this man? Actually, nothing was wrong with him. Everything was wrong with me. I was obese. This was my point—the turning point where I had to make a decision—a decision to live or die. How does one get to be 265 pounds and yet not realize they have a problem? Easily.

> *"Often it takes some calamity to make us live in the present. Then suddenly we wake up and see all the mistakes we have made."*
> *~Bill Watterson*

## Just Not Good Enough

My mom and dad believed in an honest day's work for an honest day's pay. My mom worked her way up the ranks in a retail chain by working 10-12 hours a day. My dad worked 24-hour days several days a week as a firefighter and part time as a security guard. They were both superheroes to me. Mom because she was making career moves in a male-dominated field and my dad for his tenacity and bravery.

Although I admired their character and work ethic, there were times that I wished their occupations were different.

With such hectic work schedules, my parents couldn't attend many recitals, plays, band performances or field trips. The demands of their jobs just didn't allow it. Every once in a while, they would work something out and arrange to come, but life often got in the way. I knew they loved me and I somewhat appreciated how hard they had to work to keep a roof over my head, but secretly I longed for more of their time and attention.

My young mind couldn't properly process what was going on around me, so I jumped to my own conclusions; none of them were good ones. I developed an "I'm not good enough" complex and the more time that passed, the more it got out of control. I started to think that if my parents had a choice between spending time with me and going to work, that they would always choose the latter. I was convinced that's where they wanted to be. I wasn't important enough to merit their attention; silly I know, but that's what I believed.

I felt isolated. I was an only child. There were no kids my age on my block and I saw my cousins on occasion, but not enough to make up for the loneliness I felt. I wanted so desperately to have someone to play with, someone to talk to, and someone that enjoyed my company. A hole had started forming in my heart that only grew with time. It was the beginning of looking for love in all the wrong places.

### The Introvert

I was determined to work smart, not hard and be the first in my family to earn a college degree. That degree would open the door of opportunity for me to create a better life without having to work as long and hard as my parents. I can remember dreaming out loud to my mom, dad, and aunties, explaining how I would one day be "in charge," either owning my own business or running someone else's. A degree in business was the first step.

At times it was hard for my family to reconcile my personality and my career goals. I was extremely introverted and only kept a close

2

circle of friends. I wasn't much of a talker and although people saw me as a leader, I always shied away from the limelight. On the other hand, I was very business-minded; always looking for ways to earn money. I often agreed to take on extra household chores to increase my allowance and I took a job bagging groceries at a local grocery store at age 16.

Like every teenage girl, I was into boys. For some reason, I had a thing for athletes and bad boys and was surprised when some of them expressed an interest in me. For them, there was a certain mystique to a "good girl" who didn't get into trouble and I liked how it felt to be the focus of their attention. But time after time, I was disappointed because it seemed that they were more interested in my body than they were in me. Is it too much to ask for a guy to actually be interested in *me*? I grew tired of octopus hands and the constant pressure to give in and decided to focus the majority of my energy on academics. Getting into a good college was my highest priority and I just didn't have time for games.

I re-focused on my studies and it paid off. I graduated 10th in my high school class and my teachers spoke so well of me in my letters of recommendation that I was admitted to four colleges. It was a tough decision, but I decided on Virginia Tech. It's highly competitive business program admitted me as a freshman and financial aid would cover my expenses the first year. It couldn't get any better than this.

In August of 1991, I headed for college with illusions of grandeur. I'd graduate with a degree in Finance, take my series 7 exams and secure a stockbroker job in Atlanta. I would earn a comfortable salary of $40 - $50K a year and it would only be a matter of time before the nice home and car followed. My dream didn't stop there; I'd continue to work my way up until I realized my dream of becoming CEO and somehow, in between my superwoman pursuits, I'd get married and have 2.5 kids to boot. I grew up hearing about the American dream; now I was determined to get my piece of it.

## Freedom of Choice

College was a whole new experience for me. My parents worked hard to shelter me from the evils of Richmond, but in Blacksburg the world was my oyster. I could go wherever I wanted with whomever I wanted and stay as long as I wanted. At age 17, I was completely and totally free to be me. The funny thing is I wasn't completely sure who I was. I was still a little on the shy side but slowly and surely I started opening up and getting to know other people. Soon I had a core group of friends on campus that I studied, partied, and hung out with. For the most part, I stayed out of trouble, with one exception.

I still had a thing for athletes and bad boys and ran into my share of both on campus. It probably didn't help that my dorm was directly across from the athlete's dorm. To make matters worse, my roommate dated a football player. The good girl charm was still in effect and by then, my tall, slim frame had started to fill out a little. I started enjoying the attention I received. I lost focus on my studies and it showed.

I earned my first "F" ever in statistics my freshman year and had to enroll in summer school. I considered it a wake-up call, got a tutor and started being more diligent in my studies. Despite my best efforts, Accounting and Economics kicked my butt and by the time I had gotten to my junior year, I was seriously considering changing my major from Finance to Marketing or Business Administration so I could avoid some of the advanced finance courses. I wasn't measuring up academically and I knew my dream was in jeopardy.

I called my mom to discuss my bright idea to switch majors but she didn't share my enthusiasm. She listened attentively then asked me a series of questions that revealed my underlying motives: I was afraid of failing. I didn't know if I had it in me to finish what I started. Maybe I had bitten off more than I could chew? My mom assured me that I could do whatever I put my mind to and said she didn't want to see me give up on my dream and regret it later. I didn't want to let her or myself down, so I decided against changing my major. I was going to buckle down and press my way through hoping that it would all work out in the end.

I signed up for summer school classes to lessen my per-semester course load and that made things a little more manageable. I was able to devote more time to each class and my grades started to improve. To my surprise, I survived International Finance and Investment Analysis and was on track to finish with a 2.7 GPA. Not horrible, but certainly not stellar. Getting a job as a stockbroker was probably out, but I thought I could still get a job in financial services, perhaps for a bank or insurance company. It was a hard pill to swallow, but I was proud of myself for not giving up and making the best out of a tough situation.

In the spring semester of my senior year, the job hunt began. I was still hoping to move to Atlanta and focused my job search there. I came across several job opportunities but quickly found it difficult to compete with the 3.0's and 4.0's of the world. Since none of us had any real-world experience, recruiters placed a big emphasis on grades and mine just didn't cut it. Now the kid that had always been an academic stand out was left out. I got a couple of letters of recommendation from my professors, but they weren't glowing ones like I received back in high school. I submitted resume after resume, but graduation came and went and I had no job offers. My confidence was a little shaken, but I tried to remain optimistic that I could still create a good life in Richmond. Maybe I would get a chance to move to Atlanta later.

Catch-22

Upon my return home, the old Catch-22 – can't get job without experience and can't get experience without a job – kept rearing its ugly head. It seemed as though every classified ad required at least 2 years of experience! I tried sending my resume anyway, hoping someone, anyone, would give me a chance and nothing. Friends and family tried to help, still nothing. I started to apply for any and everything – even an administrative job at the newspaper. When they offered me a job – at $16,000 a year- I thought, "No way, I didn't spend 4 years in college for this!" I declined the job offer and kept looking. I knew I could do more than my grades represented and wanted someone to give me a chance to prove it. I thought, "They just don't realize my potential."

After weeks of searching and applying with no luck, a friend of the family suggested trying a temp agency. She could tell I was getting down and shared her story of how temping had led to full-time employment. Thankful for the lead, I went to several, signed up, and finally one called! The agency said there was a job in financial services – "great," I thought, "right up my alley!" Then she said something I didn't expect, the assignment was at a storefront finance company in a retail shopping center. Wow. What a far cry from the downtown skyscraper I had envisioned. I told myself it was just temporary, I would find something else. I accepted the assignment and made up in my mind that I would keep looking. I couldn't give up a bird in the hand for one in the bush.

While I was looking for other employment, I gave the temp job all I had. I got to work on time, stayed late, and volunteered to do extra. One day, the manager pulled me aside and shared that the office had been through a string of temps that didn't work out and I was a pleasant surprise. I appreciated the compliment but had zero intention of staying. I had a dream and was bent on achieving it. I kept filling out applications and submitting resumes. Weeks went by and I didn't hear a word.

Finally the company offered me a full-time job as a management trainee – at a salary of $18,000 a year. I would go through a training program and if I did well, could one day run my own branch. From what I heard, the branch managers did pretty well salary-wise and they received a company car – a nice perk. But like my parents, they worked extremely long hours. I took the job but inwardly thought, "Thanks, but no thanks," on the branch manager gig. I would continue to explore my options.

Remaining positive was becoming increasingly difficult. I had friends that skipped college, went straight to UPS and Phillip Morris that were living large! I had given up four years of my life and incurred over $20,000 in student loan debt and my best offer was $18,000?! I couldn't believe it. I was trying to hold on to an ounce of dignity, I kept telling myself, "It's only temporary. I'll be back on track in no time."

## Looking for Love

Around this time, I met "Eric" and I thought we were a perfect match. He was tall, dark, and handsome and he was a former athlete. "Eric" was a few years my senior and was working hard to move up the corporate ladder. We got along very well and I could see us one day marrying and starting a family. But he was the type that wanted to have his cake and eat it too. "Eric" was very upfront with the fact that he wanted an open relationship, but what he really meant was that he wanted me all to himself while he played the field. I convinced myself that I was going to beat him at his game and eventually he'd come around. I thought I could play with fire and not get burnt – that I wouldn't get emotionally invested. It was a lie and I fell for it lock, stock, and barrel.

A couple of years passed and I was now 24, but my fairy tale still wasn't even close to coming true. I had left the finance company and was working in an entry level sales position for a major bank. My salary had improved some – to $24K – but I went to work each day feeling that my talents, skills and abilities weren't being fully utilized. I needed my work to be mentally stimulating and challenging and this was anything but. Once again I tried to make the best of a bad situation, but I couldn't help but feel like my career and life were at a standstill.

"Eric" and I had been so-called dating for three years but he remained very much the same. He had 50 million excuses for why he wasn't ready to commit and we should just leave things as is. It took a while, but I finally started to realize that "Eric" had no intention of settling down – at least not with me – and I had a decision to make. I could ask him to choose between them and me and risk losing him, cut my losses and walk away, or stay in the dead end relationship and deal with the emotional pain. It was apparent I attached myself to the wrong guys. Why?

A part of me still wanted to hold on thinking that having a man around some of the time was better than having no man around at all. And when "Eric" was around, I felt special. He was very charming and attentive, as if I were the only girl that meant anything to him. Clearly, it wasn't true, but during those brief moments I could pretend that it was. In my fantasyland, everything was perfect, but it never lasted. When he wasn't with me, responses to my pages were delayed and sometimes didn't come until the next day. Then I didn't feel important and my heart was torn in a million pieces. I decided I couldn't take it anymore and broke things off. While in some ways I was relieved, I was also miserable and lonely. I was an emotional mess.

## Semi-Independence

I decided that it was time for a change of scenery. A friend I had made at the bank, "Tracy," offered to let me share her apartment which was about 45 minutes outside of Richmond. We would carpool to work and split household expenses. I had vowed "no more roommates" when I left college, but hey, at least I could say I wasn't living at home! I had visited several times before and enjoyed the slower pace, community activities and lower cost of living. The area reminded me of pleasant memories I had as a kid, spending the summer in the "country" with my grandmother, aunts, and cousins. I took her up on her offer and was happy to be finally asserting a little independence.

Although the overall cost of living was lower, I was still in over my head. I was still paying on my student loans and had racked up some credit card and furniture bills from a previous failed attempt to move out on my own. My half of the rent, bills, gas and food added up quickly and eventually, I fell behind on my bills. Receiving late notices and collection calls became the norm and my stress level rose.

At this point, I felt like nothing was going right. I just wanted a way out - a way to dull the pain of my stalled career, the poor relationship choices, the mounting bills and my "not good enough" complex. Unfortunately, I started looking for comfort in all the wrong places.

Addiction to Comfort

I ate fast food a lot. This was a bad habit I picked up in my teenage years, but with the added stress, it was now 10 times worse. I ate fast food every day at lunch and sometimes for breakfast and dinner. I didn't try to eat anything even remotely healthy. I'm talking a Quarter Pounder with Cheese, fries, a soda and sometimes a milkshake!

When I wasn't eating fast food, my eating habits were no better. Although I really didn't have it to spend, I enjoyed going to nice sit down restaurants, ordering a nice big fat rib eye, baked potato with butter, and dessert. In my mind, it was a small price to pay for a momentary escape. Food was becoming a drug.

To make matters worse, every Sunday we went to "Tracy's" mom's house for dinner. I tell you, it was almost like Thanksgiving! There was always an expansive spread of food and it was all delicious. Smothered pork chops, BBQ ribs, fried fish or chicken, meatloaf. You name it, we had it and in abundance. It was not uncommon for me to come back for seconds. The funny thing is I had no thought that it would eventually catch up to me.

Over time, I developed a serious drinking problem too – no not alcohol – soft drinks. I was famous for getting a big 32 oz. cup of Mountain Dew twice a day at work. At home, I drank Kool-Aid, sweet tea and fruit juices like they were going out of style. I absolutely hated water.

In between meals, I snacked often out of stress and/or boredom. My favorites were potato chips, Doritos, Cheetos, Little Debbie Nutty Bars, Reese's cups, and Butterfingers. I loved them because they were cheap, tasty, and provided an instant feel good. It seemed like I was always hungry. My life completely revolved around food.

All of these foods and drinks were things I enjoyed as a kid, but something had drastically changed. As a child, I pretty much ate what I wanted and it had very little effect on me. But now, I started to pick up weight and fast. I didn't make the connection that I was eating junk and comfort foods in much larger quantities and I hadn't considered that my life was now completely sedentary. Sitting in a cubicle all day and not being physically active was wreaking havoc on my metabolism and I was none the wiser. I was completely oblivious to what was happening until it was too late. It seemed that one day my clothes fit a little snug and the next I ballooned to 265 pounds. I know that's not what happened, but that's how it felt. One minute I was wearing a size 8, the next a size 24W.

## Big and Beautiful

Still, I reasoned that I was not *that* big. I am a decent height for a woman – 5'9' – and because of that I didn't look as big as I was. Seating in airplanes was getting a little snug and I almost got kicked off of a rollercoaster ride because my hips were too wide, but still I wasn't *that* big. I could always find someone who was bigger and more lifeless and out of shape than I was; at least I wasn't *that* bad. You can always find someone worse off than you to justify your self-sabotaging behaviors. I wore a size 24W but there *were* bigger sizes.

On top of that, a subculture was forming. Millions across the world were tired of being ridiculed for being fat and had started to fight back. The subculture campaigned for equal rights and labeled the weight loss industry as pushers and anyone who went along as conformists. The movement contended that big was beautiful, leading to euphemisms like full-figured, plus sized, and BBW (Big Beautiful Women) designed to affirm and build the self-esteem of larger women.

As Americans' waistlines grew bigger, the mantra of size acceptance gained momentum. As a plus-sized woman, I could now choose the abbreviation BBW as my body type in personal ads and online dating services so men that preferred full-figured women could easily identify me. I was a part of an exclusive group, almost like a sorority or club. There were BBW-themed events, conferences, TV shows and websites. In the subculture, skinny was out and big was in.

In 2008, over one-third of adults were classified as obese. Once upon a time it was hard to find decent looking clothes in larger sizes but those times were no more. Plus-sized clothing was now big business and fashionable. If department stores didn't have what you were looking for, there were now specialty stores like Lane Bryant and Ashely Stewart that carried nothing but plus-sized clothing. I became desensitized to my weight problem. I thought, "Not everyone is meant to be thin."

The make-up of my family seemed to substantiate my argument. Most of the women and some of the men were overweight and had been for quite some time. Small and limber in their youth, they had each settled into bigger bodies as the years passed. Maybe it was hereditary? Something that made us genetically disposed to weight gain?

Facing the Music

The truth was that there were a lot of contributing factors to me being overweight but the biggest of which was denial. I tried to put up this façade but I felt out of control in every sense of the word.

I was in denial about:

**My career**. Truthfully, I didn't have a career plan. I had no idea what I wanted to be when I grew up and hadn't invested any time in figuring it out.

**My relationships**. I consistently chose men that were emotionally unavailable and unwilling to commit. Still, I blamed them rather than looking at the common denominator in the equation – me.

**My financial situation**. I was broke. I didn't have any money in savings. I was living from paycheck to paycheck and always ended up with more bills than money.

**My faith**. I grew up in church but I hadn't fully let church grow up in me. I hadn't matured and developed spiritually as I should have and was therefore easily deterred by the pressures of life.

**My health**. Intuitively, I knew carrying around 100+ pounds of excess weight wasn't healthy, but since I wasn't on medication and didn't feel bad, I figured all was well. There were no outward signs that I was sick, which to me automatically meant that I was okay.

**My family history**. Sickness and disease were prevalent in my family. It probably wasn't a coincidence that being overweight was also common.

**My growth**. As a child I believed I would be a leader and had all these dreams of what I would do and where I would be. But dreaming is where it stopped. I stopped reading regularly after college and wasn't challenging myself to grow my leadership skills. I just thought it would happen, by osmosis I guess.

I was in denial about a lot of things. It was easier to deny than to confront. But eventually, I would be confronted and have to make some decisions, decisions that would change my life forever.


Reflection Points:

1. What have you been in denial about?
2. How is that serving you?

# Chapter 2 – Temporary Fix

This was not my first rodeo. I had tried several times to lose weight with temporary success.

Sweet 16

I went on my first diet when I was 16. My clothes were getting a little tight and I decided that losing 10 pounds would do the trick. I checked out a teen dieting book at the library for some quick tips. What I took away from the book was that I needed to cut back on how much I ate. It provided various examples of how I could reach my goal by making a few adjustments. By shaving a couple of hundred calories off of each meal, I could reasonably expect to reach my goal weight within a matter of months. Seemed pretty straightforward, so I came up with a plan and went to work. I didn't really try to eat healthier, I just ate less food, walked 5 days a week and it worked. I started to see the scale move. I was back at my goal weight in a matter of months.

The fact that I was able to reach my goal weight without really addressing the heart of the issue probably did more harm than good, like most short cuts. Once I was happy with my weight, I started picking up some of my old eating habits. When I noticed that the scale was tipping up, I just watched my food intake a little more closely. I was able to maintain my weight and in my mind, that was success. Little did I know that this would be the first of many dieting cycles that I would find myself in.

## A Fresh Start

Between 2000 and 2005, I tried Slim Fast, Weight Watchers Online and joining a gym with a friend and none of it worked, but this time was going to be different! I had a goal, something to keep me motivated and on track: a wedding. My friend was getting married that summer and a few of us in the office decided that we would start a weight loss competition for accountability and support to ensure we reached our goal. Highly competitive at heart, I was all over it. Just like I did as a teenager, I came up with my plan and went to work.

I cut back on the quantity of food I ate and hit the gym 5 days a week. Because I lived in a rural area with no gym, that meant packing all my work clothes, toiletries and curling iron the night before, getting up at 5:00 AM, and driving 45 minutes to get to the gym. Then, after my 45 minute workout, I hit the showers and fought with my hair (no natural hairdo then) so that I would look somewhat presentable for work. I did that for a good 5 months, won the weight loss competition, and by wedding day I looked great!

I was down to 225 pounds and wearing a size 18. I received a lot of compliments and encouragement. It felt good to feel attractive again and I had every intention of keeping it up. I mean, I had laid a great foundation. They say it takes 21 days to create a habit and I had been getting up at 5:00 AM for over 150 days. "I've got this!" I thought.

## False Reality

But don't you know, with the wedding day behind me, I lost my motivation. I got tired of depriving myself. I wanted to go back to my regular fast food and junk food routine and not force myself to eat in reduced quantities. I decided I would allow a little more freedom in my diet and just keep going to the gym to "balance it out." I didn't know any better and actually believed it would work.

At first, nothing happened. I hopped on the scale each week and my numbers remained the same. This lulled me into a false state of confidence and my eating habits got progressively worse. Then I became even more deceived and decided that I could stop going to the gym and still maintain my weight. I would just take a walk a few days a week and everything would turn out okay.

It wasn't long before I quit everything and gained 10 of the 40 pounds I lost back. Instead of going back to the drawing board and figuring out where I went wrong, I considered it a sign that this was the smallest I could ever hope to be. Losing weight was a losing battle and I didn't have what it took to beat the odds and win.

> *"Fitness – if it came in a bottle, everybody would have a great body."*
> *~ Cher*

Reality Check

Looking back, there were some great lessons wrapped up in this experience:

*Traditional dieting doesn't work.*

For many people, a diet is a temporary way of being – for 30 days, 60 days, or 90 days - after which life returns to normal. All of the time and energy is focused on reaching a certain weight by a certain time and we will do just about anything to reach it.

It's not uncommon to go to extreme measures (i.e. drastic reduction in calorie intake, fat blockers, two-a-day workouts) with no thought as to how and if we can maintain it. This is a recipe for disaster because for most of us the extreme plan that we put together (i.e. eating 1,200 calories a day and hitting the gym 7 days a week) is not sustainable. We only agree to do it because we believe it's a short-term sacrifice, and that mindset is the crux of the problem. Temporary changes can only yield temporary results.

*Maintaining your weight is equally as hard as losing it.*

Many falsely assume that once they reach their goal weight, life will get easier. That somehow maintaining weight loss is easier than losing it. Ironically, that is the furthest thing from the truth.

The truth is whatever you do to lose the weight you will have to do (and then some) to maintain it. A crazy thing happens as you lose weight: your body needs less calories to function and you burn less calories during exercise. If the new smaller you were to go back to eating like the larger you used to, you will gain weight, no ifs, ands, or buts about it.

Whatever plan we create must be one that we can see ourselves doing for the rest of our lives and since life changes, our plan has to be flexible enough to handle those changes. There will be some weeks where 6 days of exercise is possible and others where it can only be 4 days. Swearing off potatoes, bread, and cookies is doable for 3 months but for most of us, it's not doable for a lifetime. Our diet (way of eating) needs to allow us an opportunity to be human and enjoy some of the foods we love, yet have sufficient structure to keep us from going overboard. And when we do mess up, because we will, we have to have a plan for how we will work our way back.

*Motivation doesn't last.*

Wanting to look good for a wedding, vacation, etc. can be temporarily motivating. The thought of walking down the aisle or beach at your current size may be overwhelming. Then there are the pictures; everyone knows the camera adds 10 pounds! That, in and of itself, is enough to get you fired up and ready to hit the gym, but will it last?

The trouble with using an event as your primary motivator is that the event will come and go. What will keep you focused when there is no event to look good for? When no one is snapping pictures?

Furthermore, a wedding, vacation, or event that is 6 months away is, well, 6 months away. While we try to plan for the future, we still have to contend with the here and now. For many of us, some arbitrary thing that is happening in 6 months isn't enough to keep us from giving into food cravings now and crawling out of bed when we just don't feel like it.

Willpower is a necessary factor in the weight loss equation. There will be times where you have to exercise your will to make the right decision when you'd rather make the wrong one. But consider this: we will make a minimum of 3 food choices per day (breakfast, lunch, and dinner), 7 days a week, 365 days a year, for the rest of our life. How likely is it, that without added motivation, we will always choose long-term benefits over short-term gratification?

We need more than will power, we need why power. We need a vision for our life that is so strong that it can bring us to tears. The thought of gaining something or losing something so dear to us that we are willing to make the painful sacrifices necessary to step out of our comfort zone and move beyond our current condition. You need clear and compelling vision to reach your goals in health and fitness and in life.

My why came at a time that I least expected it.

Reflection Points

1. Have you ever gone to extreme measures to lose weight? Why and how?
2. Rate your willpower on a scale of 1 to 10. Why do you rate it that way?

# Chapter 3 – Me? No, Not Me. Me?

> *"When we least expect it, life sets us a challenge to test our courage and willingness to change; at such a moment, there is no point in pretending that nothing has happened or in saying that we are not ready. The challenge will not wait. Life does not look back. A week is more than enough time for us to decide whether or not to accept our destiny."*
> *~ Paulo Coelho*

"Are you still in management at the bank?" the doctor asked. "Yes," I replied. "Still working a lot of hours?" I replied in the affirmative again. I felt like I was in the hot seat. I didn't know where the conversation was going, but I knew I didn't like it.

## Jekyll or Hyde?

It was December of 2007 and I had gone to the doctor for a physical exam required for grad school admission. Finally, my life seemed to be back on track. I had earned a few promotions at work, my income had increased, I had bought my own townhome, and now I wanted to take my education to the next level. On to bigger and better things!

"Tell me about the course load for this program?" I shared that we were expected to make a time commitment of about 20 hours a week. I could see him doing the math in his head. He looked at me like he couldn't believe what he was hearing. "You realize that you are a disaster waiting to happen don't you?" he said. I was thinking,

"What? No." But I was so shocked by his statement that I was incapable of uttering a word. I just sat there with a dumbfounded look on my face. I was at a loss for words.

My mind started wandering, "A disaster waiting to happen? What does he mean?" He quickly closed that gap by leading into this speech about how I was putting myself in a dangerous position. It "was only a matter of time" before I would end up "really sick or worse." "Or worse?" I thought. "What could be worse than really sick?" And then it hit me, the only thing worse than being really sick is being dead.

My mind went all over the place again. "How can this be? I feel fine." I thought. "This doctor is tripping, it can't be that bad, can it?" It turned out that it was that bad. I needed to make some changes and I needed to make them now.

Risky Business

According to the National Heart, Blood and Lung Institute,[1] there are 8 primary risk factors for heart disease:

1. High blood pressure
2. High blood cholesterol
3. Diabetes
4. Smoking
5. Being overweight
6. Being physically inactive
7. Having a family history of early heart disease
8. Age (55 or older for women)

Of the eight factors, I had three. I was overweight, physically inactive, and had a family history of early heart disease. Sadly, I was also working on number four (hypertension).

Somewhat of a blessing and a curse, my doctor also saw my mother. My mom had struggled with high blood pressure and eventually ended up on medication. He knew all about my grandfather's battle with heart disease and him eventually needing a pacemaker. Red lights were going off in his head and he was trying to warn me.

To make matters worse, I had something else working against me. Although stress is not officially a heart disease risk factor, Harvard researchers have observed a strong correlation between women's job stress and cardiovascular disease. A recent Women's Health Study[2] revealed that women in high stress jobs had a 40% increased risk of heart disease (including heart attacks and the need for coronary artery surgery), compared with their less stressed counterparts. My stress level was already high due to my work responsibilities and would only get worse with the addition of the MBA course load. He was right. I *was* a disaster waiting to happen.

On one hand I was thankful that he took the time to level with me. I had friends who told me they had just been put on medication without the doctor mentioning healthier eating and regular exercise as a viable alternative. On the other hand, I was very afraid. He had given me a gift – the opportunity to change the course of my future and make some changes so I could lead a long and healthy life. But how?

Partial Deliverance

I wanted to take advantage of the opportunity, but he didn't tell me what to do or how to do it. I needed something beyond "eat better and exercise" because I had been down that road before. I wanted him to tell me which diet to follow, which exercises I should do to get the best results, and most importantly give me a plan that would help me stay on track.

My doctor and I didn't discuss how to lose the weight in any detail. On the surface, this would seem odd. In a country where over 35% of adults are obese and at a high risk for obesity-related conditions[3] including heart disease, stroke, type 2 diabetes and certain types of cancer, you would think there would be a lot of talk in the medical community about helping patients get healthy. But even with these out-of-control numbers, research indicates[4] that the amount of time doctors spend talking to patients about health and fitness is actually decreasing rather than increasing!

I believe that there are several reasons for this:

*Insufficient Training*

In a 2009 study, just 27% of the schools met the minimum standard of nutrition training. Sadly, that is down from 38% in 2004. I'm sure each doctor has an idea of what is necessary to lose weight at a basic level but everyone is different. How do they address the nutrition needs of 10-20+ different patients a day?

*Fear of Being Charged with Malpractice*

A lack of nutrition training has led to a discomfort around the topic and a fear of giving erroneous information. Researchers contend that medical students need at least 25 hours of nutrition instruction to be adequately prepared to advise patients. According to a study published in the Journal of Academic Medicine in 2010, doctors receive an average of 19 hours of total nutrition education down from 22.3 hours in 2004. I'm not sure I would feel comfortable with those odds. In today's sue-happy culture, a piece of well-intentioned but ill-informed advice could easily result in career-ending malpractice suits.

*Doctors Are Overworked*

In the current health system, doctors are trained to see as many people as possible, as quickly as possible. Even if they did have the knowledge, taking the time to have an in-depth conversation would decrease the number of patients they see and therefore reduce their income. A lower income would significantly impact the quality of life for them and their families.

*Behavioral Counseling Hasn't Always Been Covered*

The truth is that health insurance companies really run the industry. Generally speaking, the services that are covered by insurers will be offered and services that are not will not.

Back in 2008, some insurers offered weight-loss and wellness programs, and others paid for prescription weight loss medication and expensive bariatric surgeries, like gastric bypass and gastric banding. It was completely up to the insurer whether or not they wanted to include these programs as a result, some did and some did not. With this inconsistency in practice, some patients received help and others were left to figure it out on their own.

Effective January 2014, most insurance plans will now be required to offer weight loss help,[5] but the coverage offered is completely up to the individual health care plans. The good news: patients determined to be obese will receive initial weight loss guidance and be referred to a professional service. The bad news: with no policing, plans will still vary widely in terms of the services they offer and it is very much a one-size-fits-all approach. Telephone counseling has become increasingly popular and while effective for some, a person who is 200 pounds overweight may require more face-to-face one-on-one counseling. Still this is an improvement for many patients who have been looking for some guidance and support. Under a provision of the law, some grandfathered plans still won't have to cover obesity screening, so some patients will still be left out in the cold.

### Doctors Know That Patients Need More Than They Can Give

Making a lifestyle change is no easy task. Continuous coaching and support is often required for lasting change and this is beyond the scope of a doctor's business model and training.

According to obesity researcher Donna Ryan,[6] patients are likely to lose more weight if they enroll in a comprehensive lifestyle program led by a nutritional professional than they will with just the doctor's admonition to eat less and move more.

I quickly realized that while my doctor sounded the alarm, he would not be able to guide me through the process. He gave me the clear and compelling why I needed: If I didn't change, my quality of life would be at risk or worse case, I wouldn't live at all.

I needed to find some answers and quickly, but I had no idea where to look.

## Reflection Points

1. How many times has your doctor spoken to you about losing weight?
2. How many times have you taken him or her seriously?
3. How many of the 8 risk factors for heart disease do you have?

1. Nhlbi.nih.gov, 2013

2. Health Harvard, 2013

3. CDC.gov, 2013

4. Chicago Tribune, 2013

5. USA Today, 2013

6. USA Today, 2013

# Chapter 4 – Great Ideas, But Why Am I Confused?

> *"Disenchantment, whether it is a minor disappointment or a major shock,*
> *is the signal that things are moving into transition in our lives."*
> *~William Throsby Bridges*

After I got over the shock of my doctor's office visit, I began looking for the solution to my weight problem. I decided that this time I would have to have a totally different approach. It wouldn't be about reaching a certain size by a certain time. As a matter of fact, I wouldn't set any numerical goals initially. All I knew is that I wanted to be healthy and I wanted to live a good life. (One void of medication) and talks like the one I had just received.

I knew that in order for that to happen, I would have to become more physically active. I was currently taking Tae Kwan Do classes and I loved the focus and discipline it required. I just wasn't sure it was intense enough to result in significant weight loss. It was time to weigh my options.

<u>Let's Get Physical</u>

*Power Walking*

I gained an appreciation for walking when I went on my first diet at age 16. It was simple and I found the experience to be somewhat therapeutic. I would see others of all shapes and sizes on the track, yet there was no air of superiority. Everyone was welcome and most people seemed to be in a good mood. Walkers frequently nodded or said hello when their paths crossed. The scenery was also pleasant and alluring – seeing the colorful trees, hearing the birds chirp and watching squirrels scurry by helped me to slow down and appreciate living. Best of all, it worked! I lost the 10 pounds and felt good in my clothes again.

Having had success with it in the past, I had every reason to believe power walking could work for me again. There was just one problem: I was all grown up, no longer living in my mom's house, and I didn't live across from the track anymore. My subdivision was busy with cars coming in and out and wasn't really conducive to walking. I was near a main road but only portions of it had paved sidewalks.

In a flash of inspiration, I had an idea: I could drive to one of the nearby schools and use their track. Definitely doable. Or I could power walk on the treadmill at the gym.

*The Gym*

In my most recent semi-successful attempt of losing weight for the wedding, hitting the gym 5 days a week produced some impressive results. I lost 40 pounds in 5 months and in time I went from exhausted to energetic. I finally experienced that endorphin boost I had heard so much about. With grad school right around the corner, I could use all the extra energy I could get.

The only problem was I hated the gym…literally! While effective, inside the four walls I found walking (on the treadmill) boring. The elliptical machine wasn't much better. It all felt like 45 minutes of pure torture. Then there were the weight machines and equipment. I knew I should be doing some weight training, but I never remembered how to use the machines. Perhaps, most unsettling was the feeling that I stood out like a sore thumb.

Initially, I had hoped the gym would be a place of support and camaraderie but it never felt that way to me. It felt like the gym was really a club for fit people and every once in a while a fat person was admitted. It was full of people in their tank tops and tight shorts showing off their gorgeous bodies and here I was in an oversized t-shirt and baggy sweats trying to hide mine. On occasion I noticed a disapproving look and whispering lips. It wasn't everyone, but it happened enough to make me feel out of place. I wasn't sure I wanted to endure that again.

One day while driving to work, I noticed that a new gym had opened up. The gym was called Curves and it was just for women – nice! I decided to go by and check it out. I liked that there was a structured approach to exercise that focused on exercise efficiency. The representative claimed in just 30-minutes, I could get in a quality workout encompassing every major muscle group *and* burn up to 500 calories! I liked the sound of that!

I was all ready to sign up but when I asked about the hours, my heart sank. It closed at 7 PM on weekdays, was only open a half of a day on Saturday and closed all day Sunday. I'm sure the schedule worked great for the owner(s), but it was horrible for me.

## Hiring a Personal Trainer

Not long after the disappointment at Curves, I overheard a conversation between two women, one of which had found success by working one-on-one with a trainer. I was surprised to hear that because in my mind, trainers were for the super-rich who needed to lose weight quickly (i.e. a celebrity who had just had a baby and needed to get back to her "before" figure) or those who wanted to get muscular and "buffed." I didn't realize that hiring a trainer could be beneficial for the everyday person.

After doing some research, I realized that a good trainer didn't just focus on cardio and weight lifting during the session. He or she would hold me accountable for additional workouts that I had committed to and ask about my eating habits. I didn't like the idea of accountability, but I knew that I would be more likely to follow through if I had someone asking me about it. Added motivation!

I also liked the idea of someone showing me what I should focus on during exercise and demonstrating how the equipment worked rather than me fumbling around with that on my own. If the past in any way predicted the future, that was a recipe for disaster. Maybe he or she could come up with some routines that didn't require me to waste my life away on the treadmill the whole time!

Hiring a personal trainer was very appealing. I only had one issue: the fee. It seemed that most gyms in the area charged about $50 an hour and recommended a minimum of two sessions a week. It didn't take me long to do the math - $400 a month! That was more than my car payment and I just didn't see that expense fitting into my budget.

The Diet Dilemma

While I knew that exercise was important, I also learned from past experience that how much I ate was important. I would have to find some method of portion control. Eating "less" was relative; I needed something more structured and well-thought-out. I needed a process - a road map to follow that would get me from point A to point B.

I began reflecting on the diet programs I was familiar with - either through personal experience or through word of mouth - and thought the below were worth seriously considering. Interestingly enough, all three are still popular in weight loss circles today:

*Weight Watchers*

I had tried Weight Watchers Online with a friend back in 2004. I liked the fact that I didn't have to keep up with how many calories I ate. Instead, Weight Watchers used a point system that taught you how to make healthier food choices. Foods that were full of fiber, "good carbs" and lean proteins, were assigned lower points and some of my favorite things: cookies, candy, cakes, and fast food were assigned higher points. It was subtle but an effective way of influencing your food choices.

Overall, I liked the program well enough; I just didn't know if I would stick with it. I started off really well in 2004. I entered my food into the system each day and most days I was using but not exceeding my points balance. When I did go too far, the system showed a negative balance and that encouraged me to course correct. But entering all of my food into the system daily was a chore. It was cumbersome and I wasn't sure I would maintain it.

## The Atkins Diet

I was naturally intrigued by the Atkins diet because it allowed many of the foods I loved that were big no-no's on other diet plans: butter, bacon, cream, meat, and cheese. The drawback was that most grains, dried fruits, foods with added sugar, refined carbs, juices, most snacks and sweets, were completely out. Still, I knew that if I wanted to lose weight, I would seriously have to cut back on these things anyway. Maybe it was doable?

I also liked that the program had four phases: Induction, Ongoing Weight Loss, Pre-maintenance, and Lifetime Maintenance. The Induction phase was the most restrictive, but the possibility of losing up to 15 pounds in two weeks almost made it worth it.

The fact that the program had a Lifetime Maintenance phase was encouraging. I knew that whatever I did, I needed to be able to do it for life rather than considering it a quick fix.

The Atkins diet wasn't without controversy though. Critics barked that the diet made it easy to overeat the wrong type of protein and could be high in cholesterol and saturated fat – both of which were factors attributable to heart disease.

## The Zone Diet

This diet made some pretty bold assertions: eating an anti-inflammatory diet of 30% protein, 30% fat, and 40% carbohydrates would put me "in the zone." Not only would I lose weight but by adopting this type of diet, I could literally reverse high blood pressure and heart disease. Wow! It appeared to be just what I needed. Of course, Dr. Sears, the diet's creator, doesn't come right out and claim he has found the cure for heart disease or diabetes but it's certainly implied in the success stories in his book *Enter The Zone*. Sears believed that the classic recommendation of a diet high in carbohydrates, low in protein, and fats was largely responsible for our contraction of these life-threatening diseases. I knew very little about nutrition but I did know that eating a lot of low-quality carbs had contributed to my weight gain. I wondered if Dr. Sears was right about it contributing to my borderline high blood pressure too.

What was scary about the Zone diet was its exacting measure of what to eat. The protein/fat/carbohydrate ratio was law and had to be strictly followed. If you deviated, you were no longer "in the zone." In addition, I would have to identify the "right" amount of protein intake for me based on my size, age, and activity. My protein need, in turn, controlled the amount of fats and carbohydrates I should be eating. Ugh.

While many of the elements of the Zone diet made sense, I had some serious concerns. Its critics contended that Sears's diet was anecdotally based; there were no scientific studies that proved his specific claims. Nutritionists also felt that the diet restricted carbohydrates more than necessary.

As I sat back and reflected on all of these diets and others like Jenny Craig, Nutrisystem, and South Beach, I discovered something. While they were all touted by some, there was always someone, somewhere that had something negative to say about it! On top of that, with each, I had serious doubts about my ability to maintain them beyond 2-3 months. I had made up in my mind that this time had to be different. I had to have a plan that could work for me for life, not just in the short-term.

### A Cracked Cranium

I had searched for answers only to end up more confused. Some advocated a low-fat diet. Others a low-carb diet. What was I going to do about exercise? Could I find room in my budget for the personal trainer? Would it be a worthwhile investment?

The more I thought about it, the more my head hurt. There was a "problem" with each option. I couldn't seem to find the perfect solution and I didn't know what to do! I was overwhelmed by the choices and afraid of making a mistake. I had been here before and each time I had experienced temporary success only to end up right back where I started in a few short months. I didn't want to do that again. So in classic Tamara Jackson style, I decided that since I didn't know the right thing to do, I would do nothing. I know, I know, that wasn't a good decision. I was paralyzed by fear and had made up in my mind that no decision was better than a bad decision.

I needed help sorting through all the madness; a simple eating plan and exercise routine that I could stick to. I did find it or shall I say it found me.

## Reflection Points

1. Do you have a structured workout plan? If so, is it working for you?
2. If you are on a specific eating plan, can you see yourself staying on that plan for the rest of your life?

# Chapter 5 – This Can't Be Real

"I shouldn't be doing this," I thought, but I did it anyway. Experience has taught me that it's generally not a good idea to turn on the TV when I'm having trouble sleeping. More often than not, I get sucked into the TV program and end up wide awake making it nearly impossible to drift back off to sleep. Knowing all that, I still felt compelled to turn on the TV. I guess I had looked at the ceiling as long as I could and just couldn't take it anymore.

> *"Coincidence is God's way of remaining anonymous."*
> ~*Albert Einstein*

Sleepless in Richmond

As I flipped through the channels, I came across an infomercial that caught my attention. Actually, let me be honest, it was the trainer in the fitness infomercial that caught my attention! He was very attractive, caramel complexion, with a tall, muscular build. Two words: eye candy!

Eventually, I was no longer mesmerized by his looks and actually started listening to the program. The workout was called *Hip Hop Abs* and several ladies shared testimonials about how fun the program was. They even went so far as to say that they didn't even feel like they were working out – it was more like dancing. I thought "no way!" I couldn't imagine working out being fun. Every experience I had up until that point was anything but. Could there be a better way? Could I actually lose the weight and learn to enjoy exercise at the same time? All for less than $60? I decided it was all too good to be true and that I should try and get back to sleep. It would be time to get up for work before I knew it. I wrote the phone number on the back of an envelope "just in case."

## Decisions, Decisions

About a week later I came across the envelope I had written on and my mind went back to the night I saw the infomercial. I was torn. I really liked the idea of working out at home and the concept that I could actually enjoy exercise, but would I really do it? I had never worked out at home before and didn't know if I would really stick to it.

The thought of going back to the gym was not a pleasant one. The more I thought about getting back on the treadmill and elliptical the more my heart sank. Every time I did it, it felt like watching paint dry! I tried to pass the time by watching TV or reading but I had read that the distraction could hamper my effectiveness, reducing my calorie burn. I needed something that would keep my attention and encourage me to stay focused from start to finish. I liked the idea of hiring a personal trainer, but it was "too rich for my blood" as the older generation in my family used to say.

I decided that the gym wasn't the best option for me. Although I was now only 10 minutes away, I just couldn't see myself getting up and going there every day with grad school starting soon. I knew that when life got crazy, the first thing I would let go to the way side would be the gym. I couldn't afford to let that happen again. I needed a solution that allowed me to get a workout in anytime, anywhere. The more I thought about it, the more attractive the idea of a home workout became. I decided that I would go for it. I had 30 days to try it out and return it if it didn't work and I vowed that I would do just that.

*Hip Hop Abs* arrived about a week later – I was so excited to see it on my doorstep! I immediately opened the box and found that there was an introductory DVD to orient me to all the moves. There was also a cardio workout, abs workout, strength workout, and a lower body workout. I liked the variety. There was also a schedule that told me when to do what workout. I appreciated the fact that everything was laid out for me and I didn't have to guess at it.

New Resolve

It was now mid-December and I decided that it would be better to start the program in the New Year – you guessed it, it was my New Year's resolution. I didn't see any point of starting then knowing that Christmas parties and family gatherings full of food were right around the corner. No, I would use this time to "get ready" – to get my mind right for the impending challenge – whatever that meant.

I didn't tell anyone what I was planning to do because you know how New Year's resolutions often go. It's easy to start off strong and then fizzle. To be bursting with enthusiasm about your new life in the beginning only to find yourself tired and deflated a few weeks (or even days) later. Although, I knew I needed to do this, a part of me was afraid that this would be like all the other times.

I reflected on my last doctor's office visit. It was truly one of the scariest experiences of my life. I had had brushes with death before – a tire blowing out and my car spinning out of control on highway 81, losing control of my car in the rain and ramming into the back of the car in front of me, being in the blind spot of a tractor trailer – but this felt totally different. In each of those instances, the situations were largely out of my control. I was simply the victim of circumstance and the outcome was dependent on how I reacted and I believe divine intervention. But in this situation, I would have been largely responsible for the outcome. That was a sobering thought.

My motivation was bigger than achieving a certain look or wearing a certain size. This time, I was fighting for my life. If I didn't change, the question was not only, "How long would I live," but, "What would my quality of life be?"

When Christmas day rolled around, I was reminded of what my life could look like. As I looked around the table, almost everyone there was significantly overweight, sluggish, and on some kind of medication. I then recalled how often I had received a phone call that someone in the family was sick or had been admitted to the hospital. That had happened too many times. It seemed like each time I talked to my mom, someone was sick.

I couldn't let that be my story. At least not without giving it an honest try. January 1st my new life would begin.

## Second Thoughts

"Here goes nothing!" I thought to myself as I popped in the *Hip Hop Abs* cardio DVD for the first time. I felt like a complete sucker…I had fallen for the late-night infomercial that wooed me into believing that I could lose weight and have fun doing it. As I watched the warnings and disclaimers roll, there was a verbal sparring match going on in my head. "This is a joke. It's not possible!" said one side. "Or is it?" said the other. Finally they both decided, "Who knows!" and I was left to come to a decision of my own. I decided that the only way I would find out if it worked was to try it. Quitting before I started was no longer an option. I had too much to lose now. I had to find a way to make this work.

"This isn't too bad," I thought as the workout started. "I can do this." We started out with some simple dance inspired moves that didn't leave me breathless but I could tell I would soon be working up a sweat. I was good for the first 4 or 5 minutes and then the moves started becoming more challenging. The instructor, Shaun T., was moving a little faster and I was starting to feel the pain of being out of shape. I secretly begrudged the "class" in the video. They were all smiling and slim; it didn't appear that the workout fazed them a bit. The saving grace was the instructor. Not only was he fine, but he had this engaging smile that drew you in and made you feel as though he could actually see you. And that wasn't Shaun's only endearing quality. He had a way of sensing when it was getting really tough and would either say something silly that made you laugh or look you in the eye and encourage you to hang in there with him until the end of the set. Shaun is a master motivator and he really did make working out fun!

## Hitting My Stride

I was two weeks in and starting to actually look forward to my exercise time. Maybe there was something to be said for finding a workout that you actually enjoyed? For finding someone or something that pushed your limits without going too far? Maybe this was for real.

I was on a roll, but would now have to pack my bags and head to Gainesville for a few days for grad school orientation. Once upon a time, I would have let any interruption in my normal daily life throw me off track. Not this time. Determined that I would not fall off of my workout regimen, I took the DVDs with me. I was changing.

## Reflection Points

1. What is your motivation for getting in shape?
2. When was the last time you looked forward to your workout?

# Chapter 6 – C'mon It's a White Lie

> *"We tell lies when we are afraid...afraid of what we don't know, afraid of what others will think, afraid of what will be found out about us. But every time we tell a lie, the thing that we fear grows stronger."*
> *~Tad Williams*

"220" I said. They both looked at me like they knew I was lying. I was. I actually weighed 235 pounds, but what woman is forthcoming about her weight? Thanks in part to my doctor, I had successfully completed all of the requirements for admission for grad school and was participating in a day of team-building activities. The first set of activities didn't go too well and this one was shaping up to be even worse.

## Outdoor Adventure

This time, everyone had to be picked up and carried through an obstacle course. The goal was to do it as quickly as possible because the exercise was being timed. The two "handlers" on the team decided that they would take the smallest people first to get off to a quick start. I knew that I would not be in that bunch. The embarrassment went to a whole new level when handlers decided that each of us needed to share our weight so they could put us in weight order. Obviously these guys had never heard that it's not okay to ask a woman her weight! So I did what any self-respecting, overweight, and embarrassed woman would do. I lied! I said 220. I knew they didn't buy it and that just made me want to disappear.

Unfortunately, that wasn't the only embarrassing experience of the day. The next activity was rock climbing. I watched my slimmer, fitter counterparts climb that wall like Spiderman and thought "must be nice." I had never been rock climbing, mostly out of fear of looking like a fool. And look like a fool I did! I couldn't get a tight grip on the rocks. My hands and feet kept slipping; I fought to stay on the wall. I was sweating like crazy and exhausted from being out in the hot sun. I was determined to keep trying. I barely made it a quarter of the way up the wall before completely losing my grip and falling. The team tried to be supportive, but I couldn't help but feel like I had failed to pull my weight once again, literally.

As if that wasn't enough, the faculty and staff had one more fun-filled surprise for us – a tightrope exercise. I thought to myself "there is no way!" I couldn't imagine that I at 220, um 235 pounds, would make it safely across that rope. I toyed with a cop out—saying that I was afraid of heights—which would allow me to bow out gracefully. I was tempted, but for the sake of my team, I decided that I had to at least try. I decided to let a bunch of people go ahead of me to give me some time to work up my nerve. Finally, I couldn't put it off any longer. It was my time to go up.

I took a deep breath and began climbing up the pole. I reached the top and made the classic mistake of looking down. Why did I do that? I was completely and totally petrified. A few of my classmates were below cheering me on and encouraging me to take that first step. I wanted so badly to turn around and climb back down that pole but instead I stepped out onto the tight rope. My legs started shaking like crazy. I put one foot in front of the other like the instructor said, but it sounded much easier than it was. With every step I had to fight to keep my balance. The further I got away from the starting pole the more I shook.

The pole at the end seemed so far away. I felt so heavy on that rope, like once again my weight was holding me back. I made it a little less than halfway across before totally losing my balance and falling off the rope. Thanks to my harness, I didn't end up a splat on the ground, but my ego had taken more blows in one day than it had in 8 years of being overweight.

## Odd Woman Out

I had never felt so alienated and limited by my weight. I guess it's kind of crazy considering that 235 pounds was the lightest I'd been in six years, but it was now clear to me that there were things I could not do in the shape I was in. Still, if that had been the only consequence, the situation may not have bothered me as much. What really got to me was my inability to perform at a high level – not being able to keep up with my peers – and feeling like an outsider.

Before that day, I thought being bright, driven, and having a nice personality was enough…that I was being judged by who I was as a person, not how I looked. But was that really true? While many people were genuinely supportive during the team building activities, not everyone was. There were a few critical looks, some rolling of the eyes, and even some snickering. There were several times that I felt like the entertainment of the day. I could almost imagine them saying, "watch her make a fool of herself, what a joke!"

As the saying goes, a bad apple can spoil the whole bunch. The small group of people that poked fun at my expense stood out in my mind. I began to question other things. Was my weight impacting more than my health and physical capabilities?

## Social Stigma

In 2008, the Rudd Center for Food Policy and Obesity at Yale published a study in the International Journal of Obesity. The study, designed to investigate the extensiveness and types of self-reported weight/height discrimination in contrast to racial and gender discrimination, uncovered the following:

*Key Study Findings*

- Women were twice as likely to report daily or lifetime discrimination due to weight/height as men.
- Obese women were 1.6 to 3 times more likely to report weight/height discrimination than obese men.
- ¼ of the African-American women respondents reported weight/height discrimination, the highest of any group.
- Weight/height discrimination ranked as the 3rd most prevalent cause of perceived discrimination among women (after gender and age discrimination), and the 4th most prevalent form of discrimination reported by all adults.
- While men were not at serious risk for discrimination until they reached a BMI of 35 or higher, women experienced a notable increase in weight/height discrimination risk at a lower BMI level of 27.

*Reported Impacts*

- Almost 60% of participants reporting weight/height discrimination experienced employment-based discrimination (for example, not hired for a job) on average four times during their lifetime.
- Approximately a 1/3 of respondents reported other forms of employment discrimination such as being turned down for a job or a promotion.
- Being treated with less respect and or as inferior (for example, not as smart, not as good as others) was the most common type of daily interpersonal weight/height discrimination. About 1/3 of respondents experienced this "Often or Sometimes."
- Obese adults aged 45–54 and those in sales and clerical professions were at additional risk for weight/height discrimination.
- In some cases, weight/height discrimination was reported even more frequently than age or gender discrimination.

Sadly, studies show that the struggle isn't just in workplace equality.

Researchers contend that negative perceptions of obese people exist in health care settings – even among those that specialize in the treatment of obesity. In one study,[7] 50% of doctors believed that overweight patients were "awkward, ugly, weak-willed and unlikely to comply with treatment" and 24% of nurses said they were repulsed by their obese patients. What an arduous thought, the very ones that are counseling people to get healthy have biases against them. I bet this at least partially explains the obese person's reluctance to seek medical care.

Studies also found low opinions of the overweight and obese in educational environments. 28% of teachers in one study[8] said that becoming obese is "the worst thing that can happen to a person." Researchers Canning and Mayer scrutinized the school records and college applications of over 2500 high school students[9] and found that obese students were substantially less likely to be accepted to college despite having equivalent application rates and academic credentials to their non-obese peers. Furthermore, obese women faced lower acceptance rates than men – 31% and 42% respectively.

Before you decide that this is a 2008 problem, consider this: In 2013, the Rudd Center for Food Policy and Obesity at Yale University published a new study[10] that examined the propensity of jurors to show bias against overweight defendants. While female jurors (regardless of size) displayed no bias, men – especially lean men – were far more likely to render a guilty verdict on an overweight woman and were quicker to label her a repeat offender with an "awareness of her crimes." Weight stigma is everywhere and no one seems to care about it.

Too Close for Comfort

I had to wonder: Was I the victim of weight discrimination? Or at the very least prejudice?

I guess I'll never know for sure, but I had to acknowledge at least two areas where things were not going as I expected.

*Career*

- I had applied for several promotions and each time received unsatisfactory, vague explanations for why I didn't receive the job.
- After being turned down for promotions I felt I earned, I wasn't as confident in my abilities as I should have been and...
- I found myself holding back on sharing ideas for fear that they weren't good enough and wouldn't be considered.

*Relationships with Men*

- To the guys I was attracted to, I was a good "friend" and cool to hang out with, but I wasn't dating material.
- In the online dating space, some guys would think I was a great catch *until* they saw a full body picture.
- As a result of not being able to attract the guys I wanted, I felt I had to choose from what was available - guys that would rather play the field than commit.

This one experience led to a flood of emotions. It had surfaced some things that I wasn't sure I was prepared to deal with. Things I had been running from for a long time.

## The Scarlet Letter

Everyone has vices and imperfections, but not all are tangible or visible. A woman who cheats on her husband, has a bad temper, or is a nag cannot easily be distinguished from one who does not until you spend some time with her. A woman who is overweight or obese walks around with a scarlet letter over her head. Regardless of her true condition, the assumption is that she is lazy, less competent and lacking in self-discipline. Everyone sees her problem and judges the root cause, but no one knows her story or sees her struggle.

No one could see all of the times I had tried and failed. They just saw where I was at that point in time. And even though I wasn't making an effort to eat healthier and exercise, I could have been. How often do people look at the woman who is 100 pounds overweight and scoff, not realizing that she eats healthy, hits the gym 5 days a week and has already lost 50 pounds? It's just not fair.

Still, I am glad it *all* happened. It served as a reinforcement of my point - a painful reminder of what I had to do. I needed to be confronted with the reality of my situation so that I couldn't bury my head in the sand anymore. It wasn't about fitting in, but instead it was about standing out.

It was time for me to become the person I was born to be. It was time for me to reclaim my mind, my body, and my life. This time, I was going to do it, for good.

Reflection Points

1. How many times have you lied about your weight?
2. Do you feel as though you have been discriminated against because of your weight? How did that make you feel?
3. Are you truly living your best life?

7. ABCNews.go.com, 2013

8. Onlinelibrary.wiley.com, 2012

9. Onlinelibrary.wiley.com, 2013

10. ABCNews.go.com, 2013

# Chapter 7 – This is Just Wrong!

> *"We all want progress, but if you're on the wrong road, progress means doing an about-turn and walking back to the right road; in that case, the man who turns back soonest is the most progressive."*
> *~C. S. Lewis*

It had been 30 days since I started my new fitness regimen. The workout calendar reminded me that it was time to weigh myself again, redo my measurements, and take a new photo. This would be one of many "after" photos that would be used to tell the story of my transformation. As I contemplated jumping on the scale, I felt good about it. I was certain that my efforts would be rewarded.

## All In

For the first time, I had truly been all in and had given everything I had each and every day that I popped in the DVD. It was hard at first because I was so out of shape, but I persevered and it eventually got easier. Not only that, but I had actually been consistent with the workouts. No on again, off again this time. I did run into a few snags here and there, having gotten home later than expected, but dragging and tired, I forced myself to still get those workouts in. Each time I felt good that I didn't let my circumstances win. I did, however, decide to make some adjustments. It had become clear that evening workouts were just too risky with my schedule. Things often popped up that got me off kilter – a fire drill at work, being invited to attend an event with a friend, and sometimes, I was just plain too tired after a long day's work. I decided to move my workouts to mornings so that I could be sure I would get them in each day without interruption.

Moving my workouts to mornings was no easy adjustment. Although I felt my energy levels were highest in the morning, I didn't particularly like to get up early. I already was in the habit of pressing snooze a couple of times before getting up and wondered how in the world I would be able to pull this off. Getting up 45 minutes earlier meant the alarm would no longer go off at the usual 6:30 AM. The new time was 5:45 AM. Ugh. But this was important, so 5:45 AM it was.

The first few days under the new 5:45 AM time were a struggle. In classic Tamara Jackson style, I still hit snooze a few times and a couple of days I was a few minutes late for work. Knowing that could not continue I accepted that I had to make yet another adjustment: I would have to go to bed an hour earlier. Staying up until 11:00 – 11:30 PM and expecting to be in the mood to rise and shine at 5:45 AM just wasn't working. I needed to go to bed by 10:30 PM so that I got my 7 hours. For a few days, it was tough for me to adjust to going to bed earlier – old habits are hard to break – but I kept at it and eventually adjusted.

The Voice

After all of these adjustments and sacrifices, I felt confident that I had lost at least 5 – 8 pounds. I took a deep breath and jumped on the scale. A little nervous, I closed my eyes. "Please let this be at least 5 pounds!" I thought. I wasn't looking for a quick fix. I just wanted some encouragement that this time really could be different. I wanted to know that hard work really does pay off. I wanted to know that I could change.

I opened my eyes and looked down at the numbers on the scale. I was horrified by what I saw "234.8". "What?!" I thought. I couldn't believe it! I had worked out 6 days a week for 4 weeks, made changes to my sleeping patterns and my morning start time and nothing. Nothing! I had not lost one single pound. I was heartbroken.

At this point the "see, I told you this wouldn't work" voice kicked in. I was reminded of all the other times I had tried and failed. According to the voice, this was just another notch on the belt. I was a hopeless cause. It was out of my control. This was just meant to be. Losing weight was too hard and I was a failure. I should just send back the DVDs and get my money back.

Unfortunately, this voice and I had a long history. When I applied for jobs and didn't get them, tried new things and struggled to "get it", went to functions and didn't immediately fit in, my self-critic instantly went to work. And sadly, more often than I would like to admit, I gave in. I concluded that whatever I was trying to do or pursue was too hard and settled for plan B.

But this time was different. Something welled up within me. I didn't want my money back! I wanted this to work! I had come too far and given up too much. I can't turn back now. The scale didn't move, but I had lost a few inches. I was starting to feel more alive. My energy levels had improved and I noticed that I was able to think clearer at work and in my studies. I was getting stronger too. The first week I could only use 3 pound weights, now I had progressed up to 5 pound weights. I was making some progress; I just wasn't getting all of the results I wanted.

> *"Failure is an inside job. So is success. If you want to achieve, you have to win the war in your thinking first. You can't let the failure outside you get inside you."*
> *-John Maxwell*

### Failing Forward

Instead of giving up, I resolved that I needed to go back to the drawing board and figure out where I went wrong. I wasn't a failure, but I had failed to reach my goal. I had to step up and accept responsibility.

Somehow, someway, I missed something along the way. I had the exercise portion down, but was that the only piece of the equation?

For a reason, I can't explain, I decided to pull the *Hip Hop Abs* box out of the closet to see if there was something in there that I had overlooked. It turned out that I had. At the very bottom of the box was this small cardboard, legal sized brochure. Intrigued, I opened the guide and began to read.

I read the previously overlooked guide from cover to cover and realized that the DVDs and instructor weren't at fault. It was all me.

I had to accept 100% responsibility and it was time for more adjustments.


Reflection Points

1. Think back to a time when you did not get the results you expected and gave up. How would the outcome have been different if you had taken 100% responsibility for the ultimate outcome?
2. What is "the voice" in your head telling you?

# PART II: OXYGEN

"Happiness is not an accident. Nor is it something you wish for.
Happiness is something you design."
~Jim Rohn

# Chapter 8 – I Found Answers

It felt like blinders were being removed from my eyes. As I read the "6 Steps to Transform Your Body," I was amazed by how simple it seemed. No rocket science here. Everything was laid out in simple-to-understand terms – the complete opposite of what I had been exposed to in the past. I'll admit I was a little skeptical but still my excitement overpowered my fears. I could do this. Maybe I had finally found the blueprint to lose the weight and keep it off for good?

> *"You need to make a commitment, and once you make it, then life will give you some answers."*
> ~*Les Brown*

The approach outlined in the two-sided, blue and white brochure challenged me to look at everything I had been doing differently. I had done some things right, but there was a lot I wasn't doing. Evidently the things I hadn't been doing were hampering my results. The brochure gave me a formula, a structure that I could follow and have confidence that I would succeed. It wouldn't be easy, but if I was willing to do the work, I could see results beyond my wildest dreams. The best part was that I wouldn't have to starve myself to do it. This was a plan that was doable for life. Just what the doctor ordered!

The Formula for Success

The "6 Steps" revealed that while exercise was a crucial piece of the weight loss equation, I had overestimated its benefits. I thought that being more active allowed me to eat whatever I wanted. I was working so hard, surely I would still come out ahead! But as I read the guide, it became apparent that in order to lose weight, those "extra" calories I burned during exercise had to remain, well extra. Until that day, I had no idea that weight loss was a scientific formula...that there was an equation that was always in play that would determine whether or not I would reach my goals. I was shocked to learn that it wasn't just a matter of being more active than I used to be. No, if I wanted to lose weight, I had to hit a predefined target. I needed to create what was called a calorie deficit by reducing my calorie intake (food), increasing the number of calories burned (exercise), or a combination of both.

This was surprising to me because I had never heard weight loss explained in these terms. Whenever I had asked someone how they lost weight, their answer seemed so subjective. I "cut back on my portions," "stopped drinking so much soda," and "started exercising," "Great, I can do that!" I thought. But how much did I need to cut back? Why was soda the enemy? How much is enough exercise? I didn't know the answer to any of these questions and so I just did what I thought was right and hoped for the best. At times it worked and in others it didn't and I could never seem to put my finger on why. Now it all made sense. I didn't have to guess anymore. There was a formula and if I followed it, I would be successful.

The formula was this:

**Calories Burned – Calories Eaten = Calorie Deficit**

The brochure explained that in order to lose 1 pound of fat, I needed to create a 3,500 calorie "deficit." I was familiar with the term deficit from my economics classes. A deficit was created when government spending exceeded revenues received from taxes. This excess spending was generally financed by borrowing through the issuance of treasury bonds that eventually had to be repaid, with interest. The only difference was that in this example, we weren't talking about spending dollars, but calories. If I burned (spent) more calories than I took in, my body would have to "borrow" calories from my excess body fat to fuel my daily activities. The only difference was that in this economy, I didn't have to pay it back!

| Goal in Pounds | Calorie Deficit Required per Week | Calorie Deficit Required Per Day (Avg.) |
|---|---|---|
| 0.5 | 1750 | 250 |
| 1 | 3500 | 500 |
| 1.5 | 5250 | 750 |
| 2 | 7000 | 1000 |

I loved to research and I was so intrigued by what I read that I decided to Google "calorie deficit" to learn more. I noticed a trend – in order to lose weight safely and lessen the risk of gaining it back, it was recommended that you aim to lose an average of 1-2 pounds of fat per week. At first the 1-2 pounds a week goal sounded modest, but then I got to thinking. Within a month's time, I could lose as much as 8 pounds and in 6 months, nearly 50 pounds. Now, that's what I call motivation!

Although I was excited by what I read, I decided that once again, I would do things differently than I had in the past. Before, I had set extreme goals like losing 10-15 pounds in one month only to be disappointed when I didn't reach it. This time, I wouldn't set a specific goal in pounds. I would focus on doing the right things and trust that the right results would follow. I wouldn't pressure myself but understanding the possibilities motivated me to want to get my act together. Now that I could clearly see how it all worked – that it wasn't luck of the draw or guesswork – I had a greater level of confidence that I could really lose the weight and bypass blood pressure medication (or worse).

## A Deeper Dive

Now that I was beginning to understand the concept of a calorie deficit, I decided it was time for me to get a better understanding of calories. I had always thought that calories were inherently bad. Everyone seemed to talk about them as if they were to be avoided or minimized at all costs. But what I read in the guide made it sound as if calories were important; something that our bodies needed. Sure, it was possible to go overboard and consume too many of them, but it was now becoming clear that there was a balance. I couldn't afford to go too low or go too high if I wanted my body to function properly.

As I continued my research I learned that calories weren't bad at all. They were simply units of energy that our bodies use to perform daily activities such as pumping blood, breathing, movement, digestion - just as our cars require fuel (gas) in order to operate. The total energy required to accomplish basic functions while the body is at rest is called the body's basal metabolic rate (BMR).[11]

According to the Mayo Clinic,[12] an individual's BMR is based on three important factors:

- Body size and composition. Bigger and/or more muscular bodies burn more calories, during exercise and even at rest.
- Sex (gender). Sorry ladies, men usually have less body fat and more muscle than we do so even at the same age and weight, they'll likely burn more calories.
- Age. As we age, we lose muscle and fat accounts for more of our weight, slowing down our metabolism.

I found it interesting that being bigger actually worked to my advantage early on. It explained a lot though. Now it made sense why I was able to drop the 40 pounds so quickly in 2006. Because I was heavier, I burned more calories when I was sleeping, lying on the couch, and sitting at my desk at work. The calories I burned during exercise were also higher simply because I weighed more. How enlightening.

With all this newly found information, I decided it was time to look up my BMR. There was no way to know what it was exactly without expensive tests, but I could track down an estimate using an online calculator. As a 33-year-old female weighing 235 pounds, my estimated BMR was 1835 calories. This 1835 would go on the left side of the equation under "calories burned".

### 1835 - Calories Eaten = My Deficit

> **Quick Tip**
> To get an estimate of your basal metabolic rate (BMR), you can use an online BMR calculator like the one available at www.calculator.net.

The next piece was estimating my calories burned through daily physical activity. By definition, BMR only estimated my calorie burn at rest and although I was mostly sedentary, daily activities like reading, walking around, watching TV, and even digesting food burned calories. Then there were the calories I burned exercising 6 days a week. The question was how much did all of this contribute?

Many of the websites I visited recommended multiplying my BMR by an activity factor to derive my daily caloric need (i.e. calories burned) at my current weight. It was recommended that I choose a factor that "best suited my lifestyle", but I had a difficult time determining which one that should be. The options were:

- If you are sedentary (little or no exercise) : BMR x 1.2

- If you are lightly active (light exercise/sports 1-3 days/week): BMR x 1.375

- If you are moderately active (moderate exercise/sports 3-5 days/week): BMR x 1.55

- If you are very active (hard exercise/sports 6-7 days a week) : BMR x 1.725

- If you are extra active (very hard exercise/sports & physical job) : BMR x 1.9

While in most instances I was exercising 6 days a week, I was pretty sure *Hip Hop Abs* didn't qualify as "hard exercise". Even if I took a more conservative approach and multiplied my BMR by the moderately active factor of 1.55, the result – an average of 2,844 calories burned per day - seemed like too much. This would mean that my typical daily activities - 50 minutes of low-impact aerobic exercise, showering and getting dressed, going to and from work, sitting at my desk, eating, and doing homework - burned an additional 1,000 calories a day! Then I read the fine print and it began to make sense. Multiplying the BMR by an activity factor was only designed to serve as a *starting point*. I was to monitor my results (or lack thereof) and make adjustments as needed because my actual numbers could be significantly lower than the estimates. I didn't like the sound of that. I could envision being sorely disappointed yet again and I didn't know if I could take another blow like that.

I made an executive decision to "play it safe" and estimate my caloric burn as my BMR plus what I believed I was burning during exercise. My rationale was simple. First, the BMR calculation was already an estimate and according to what I read, could be off by 10% or more. Additionally, I had a low degree of confidence in the activity factor, especially since I was very sedentary with the exception of the time I spent exercising. To top it all off, the other piece of the equation (calories eaten) was also an approximation; in some instances the nutritional information for the foods I was eating was not available. There was a lot of estimating going on and I feared overestimating. Granted, this made my starting point slightly less scientific, but I was willing to live with that. I would rather low ball it a little and loose more weight than I expected than use the higher number and potentially face another disappointment. Regardless of the route I chose, it would be an estimation, so I decided to take a little creative license. As long as I felt the end result was manageable I figured no harm, no foul. I could always backtrack if needed. Now I just needed to estimate the calories burned during exercise.

---

**Quick Tip**

While I was comfortable using BMR + Exercise as my starting point, I urge you to do what feels right for you. At the end of the day, this is *your* journey and no one else's. Know that no calculation is perfect; you can always make adjustments later.

---

Prior to starting my research, I believed that because I was sweating and out of breath at the end of every workout, I had to be burning off an entire meal and then some! That was the rationale I used to enjoy a burger and fries and still think I could come out ahead. But the information uncovered on the Mayo Clinic website made it clear that body size and composition, age, and gender played a part. As I continued my research, I learned that my exercise ritual was also a crucial piece of the equation.

Expending Energy

According to the 2008 Physical Activity Guidelines for Americans,[13] calories burned through aerobic exercise have three additional components:

- Intensity, or how hard a person works to do the activity. All other things being equal, the individual that works harder during exercise will burn more calories. A person walking briskly (moderate intensity) will burn more calories than someone walking at a leisurely pace and a person running at 6 miles per hour (vigorous intensity) will expend more calories than the person that is taking a brisk walk.

- Frequency, or how often a person does aerobic activity. The more often you perform a task, the more efficient you become at it. A person that has been running for 5 years will burn fewer calories than someone who has just started. For this reason, we experience the biggest gains when we move from a sedentary lifestyle to an active one or continue to challenge ourselves to increase our level of fitness.

- Duration, or how long a person does an activity. Generally speaking, the longer a person exercises the more total calories they burn. If two women that are the same age and weight decide to go for a swim but one swims for 15 minutes and the other for 30 minutes, the woman that swam for 30 minutes will burn more calories (assuming she maintains sufficient intensity).

*Note: The 2008 Physical Activity Guidelines for Americans are still the most recent guidelines.*

Again, things started to make sense. When I lost weight before, I was pushing myself extremely hard in the gym. There was a display that showed me the approximate calories I was burning as I exercised based on my heart rate. The more I pushed, the more I saw that number climb. Eager for better results, I watched the people around me and noticed them increasing the incline and resistance, stepping higher and faster, and swinging their arms, and I followed suit. Being the goal-oriented person that I am, I started setting goals for my workout at the gym. Initially, my daily target was 500 calories and I did whatever was necessary to hit that number. As my level of fitness improved, I challenged myself to do more and eventually averaged 700 calories. I also made some adjustments to my diet. I didn't really eat better food, but I ate a little less. Without really knowing how I was doing what I was doing, I was able to accomplish a major feat. But, because I didn't know how or why it worked, I also struggled to maintain it. I had just been fortunate.

Since I was now using a workout DVD, I didn't have a way of estimating how many calories I was burning unless I purchased a heart rate monitor with a calorie counter. I wasn't yet ready to make that type of investment, so I decided to guesstimate how many calories I burned using an online calculator like WebMD's "Fit-O-Meter." I entered my information and it returned a number much lower than I expected --- 445 calories.

## (1835 BMR + 445 Exercise) – Calories Eaten = My Deficit

Now I had to put my thinking cap on. After doing the math, I estimated that I averaged 2,280 calories burned *on the days I worked out.* This meant I averaged about 2,280 calories burned Monday through Saturday but on Sunday (my rest day) I estimated my calorie burn was closer to my BMR (1835). Sure there was some physical activity, but not much to speak of and again I was all about playing it safe. This brought my weekly average down to 2,216. Then it hit me, since I hadn't lost any weight in the last 30 days, my "calories eaten" number had to be pretty close to my actual calories burned (which I estimated to be around 2,216 calories a day) in order for my deficit to equal zero. Ouch!

## (1835 BMR + 381 Average Daily Exercise) –  2,216 = 0

At first I thought I had made some sort of mistake in my calculations but then I thought about it. Instead of cutting back, at best case I ate about the same as before I started exercising. On more occasions than I'd like to admit, I ate more thinking that I could afford to. I had "killed it" during my morning workout, so surely I had some wiggle room, right? Wrong! I was ignorant to the facts and paid the price for it. It was now painfully clear: I had been overestimating how much exercise was doing for me and underestimating how much I was eating.

Duh

Looking back, what's funny is that I started out exploring Weight Watchers, the Atkins diet and the Zone diet as potential options, but quickly tossed them to the side and decided to do my own thing. I had decided to wing it and assumed that all would work out in the end. Now I know what a huge error in judgment that was! As mom would say, "Hope is not a strategy," she was right.

> *"Don't take the casual approach to life. Casualness leads to casualties."*
> ~*Jim Rohn*

After uncovering all of this valuable information, I realized that getting to a healthy weight would require a combination of exercise and eating better. I had to go back to the drawing board and revamp my eating habits. Habits that started in my childhood.

Once again, the little cardboard brochure would cause an epiphany.

Reflection Points

1. What is your BMR?
2. How many calories would you estimate you are burning through exercise?
3. What will you use as your starting point?

11. Unm.edu, n.d.

12. Mayo Clinic, 2013

13. Health.gov, 2008

# Chapter 9 – I Think I'm Happy

> *"It is by choices and not by chances that we change our circumstances."*
> *~Nadia Sahari*

For years food was my comforter. Had a rough day at work? Pick up a Quarter Pounder with Cheese combo from McDonalds. Tired and didn't feel like cooking? Run through the drive through at KFC. Stressed about grad school admissions? Ben and Jerry's Double Chocolate Fudge Brownie to the rescue! Bored? Crunch on some Cheetos or potato chips. Food became the constant; the one thing I could always count on to be there for me. I had become dependent upon it and used it as a tool to navigate the pressures of life. The problem was it was causing more harm than good. I needed to break free. The question was "how"?

<u>Fresh Eyes</u>

The guide had an interesting perspective on this: question everything you eat. What a novel concept. I was good at asking myself what I had a taste for, but asking questions to determine what was good for me, not so much. I knew the foods I chose to eat weren't exactly healthy, but I didn't think they were horrible either. How could they be? I wasn't the only one eating like this. Fast food, junk food, and comfort food were commonalities in my circle, so it couldn't be that bad, right? Wrong again.

I quickly learned that for long-term success – weight loss and weight maintenance – a combination of regular caloric expenditure (exercise) and caloric restriction (reduced intake) would be required. I couldn't do one without the other. I needed to do both. I was now pretty consistent with the exercise and actually enjoyed it. Now I needed to reduce my caloric intake from the 2,200 level to at least the 1,700 level to lose 1 pound a week. If I wanted to expedite my results, I'd need to cut even further.

| Goal in Pounds | Calorie Deficit Required per Week | Calorie Deficit Required Per Day (Avg.) |
|---|---|---|
| 0.5 | 1750 | 250 |
| **1** | **3500** | **500** |
| 1.5 | 5250 | 750 |
| 2 | 7000 | 1000 |

**Calories burned – Calories Eaten = Calorie Deficit**

**2,216 a day - 1,700 a day = 516 a day**

**516 a day * 7 days a week = 3,612 a week**

I'd had time to assess what went well and what didn't go so well over the last 30 days and now it was time to decide what I was willing to do about it. Willing is the key word here. I had to be honest with myself. Although I was committed to making changes, I was still very conflicted. I realized that there is often a distinct difference between what I'd *like* to do in theory and what I was *willing* to do in real life. The differentiator – the 6 letter word that separates the two - is action. If I am honest, my actions don't always line up with my intentions. I hate it, but it's true.

> *"The first and best victory is to conquer self."*
> ~Plato

## These Are My Confessions

A great example of the conflict between theory and reality is my desire to be debt-free. I realize the hold that debt has over me, putting a lock on future dollars that I haven't even earned yet. I know having debt limits my job options because I need to earn a certain amount of money to pay the bills. I'd like the benefits, the freedom of being debt free, but am I willing to make the sacrifices to get there? Truthfully, some days I am and some days, I'm not. I'm still a work in progress. Although I can see the benefits of being on the other side, I would have to give up some things that I enjoy now to achieve that goal in the future. I can't go shopping on a whim, eat out all the time, and go to every event that comes through town and accomplish my goal. It's not fun to "miss out" when others are enjoying "the good life." So, although I've made a lot of changes in my budget, there are some things that I know I could and maybe should cut that I haven't. Why? Because as much as I want or would like to be debt-free, I'm not willing to give up everything right now and I know it. There was no point in signing up for something I knew I wouldn't stick to. It would have looked great on paper. The time needed to reach my goal would be much shorter and who doesn't want to get there fast? But, it wouldn't have been realistic based on where I am right now. I'm striving, but I know I'm not there yet, so I won't put myself through the wringer by creating unrealistic goals. Instead, I called a meeting with myself and decided on a comfortably uncomfortable goal, knowing that I would build from there. I would encourage you to do the same.

> *"Successful people ask better questions, and as a result, they get better answers."*
> ~Tony Robbins

Quality Questions

There are three questions that must be answered before making a commitment to a weight loss plan, or any other goal:

1. ***Am I willing to pay?*** Make no mistake, success requires sacrifice. Over the years I had taken my share of "short cuts," and in the end the success was only temporary. Wisdom reminds us: "Easy come, easy go, but steady diligence pays off." If you're serious about changing your life, don't take short cuts, figure out what it's going to cost you to get from point A to point B the right way and then go to question 2.

2. ***How much am I willing to pay?*** We all need transportation, but there is a difference in the payment on a $5K car vs. a $50K car. Your goal must align with what you are willing to invest. You can't reach a luxury vehicle goal on an economy car budget. Wisdom says: "But don't begin until you count the cost. For who would begin construction of a building without first calculating the cost to see if there is enough money to finish it?" I had jumped in headlong into a variety of weight loss plans in the past with no consideration for what it would cost me and if that was realistic. Not this time.

3. ***How long am I willing to pay?*** Short-term commitments yield lesser results than those made for the long term. For example, saving $100 a month for 12 months = $1200 but save the same amount for 5 years and you have $6K. Here is the thing: we can't say we want the $6,000 and not be willing to commit to being disciplined for 5 years. The Good Book testifies that discipline is never pleasant at the time but it later produces a harvest for those that were willing to yield to it. We reap what we sow; we must sow discipline and restraint in the short term in order to reap prosperity and abundance in the long term - no exceptions. If I wanted to get it right this time, I would have to sign up for something that I was willing to do *for life*. Not for 60 days, 6 weeks, or even 6 months. It had to be forever and forever is a mighty long time.

It dawned on me that in the past I had bitten off more than I could reasonably chew at the time. I wanted the benefits that going hard core would produce, but I wasn't there physically, emotionally, or spiritually so I burnt out easily. Now I had a choice to make. I could take a slow and steady approach, make this change a lifestyle, and eventually get to where I wanted to be *and stay there*. Or I could let this attempt be a diet just like all the others.

### Comparison: Dieter (person A) vs. Lifestyler (person B).

### Pounds Lost/Gained Per Month

|          | A   | B   |
|----------|-----|-----|
| Jan      | -4  | -6  |
| Feb      | -4  | -6  |
| Mar      | -4  | -6  |
| Apr      | 4   | -6  |
| May      | 6   | -6  |
| Jun      | 0   | -6  |
| Jul      | -4  | -6  |
| Aug      | -4  | -6  |
| Sep      | -4  | -6  |
| Oct      | 4   | -6  |
| Nov      | 6   | -6  |
| Dec      | 4   | -6  |
| Year End | 0   | -72 |

They say that insanity is doing the same thing over and over again and expecting different results. I was tired of being insane. I wanted this time to be for real. If I wanted different results, I was going to have to do things differently.

It was hard to admit that I wasn't yet who I would like to be, but at the same time it was refreshing. In doing so, I gave myself permission to be less than perfect. I acknowledged that I was human and looking back, I believe that was the first step to lasting change.

Now that I had been honest about where I was, I could begin again more intelligently. I could create a realistic plan with some "grace" built in and build from there. And, if I stuck with it, if I was patient with myself, I would eventually reach my destination. I may not get there as fast as I'd like or as fast as my friend or co-worker did, but I would get there. Isn't that what's really important?

> *"You cannot change your destination overnight, but you can change your direction overnight."*
> ~Jim Rohn

New Direction

Armed with this new found outlook, I decided to take a moderately aggressive approach. I would aim for 6 pounds of weight loss a month, which meant that I would need to stick to about 1,500 calories per day (or move more to compensate). This was 300 calories higher than the minimum recommended calories for weight loss (1,200 calories per day) and based on my research, it was doable. It would still require me to give up some things, but not nearly as much as an extreme diet would have.

I then began answering the three questions and developing my plan:

## GOAL SETTING WORKSHEET

1. *Decide on a 30-day goal and why it's important.* Note: If your why isn't powerful enough to make you hit the gym when you'd rather relax or pass on your favorite dessert, it needs some work!

   Lose 6 pounds so that I am on track to reach a healthy BMI (Body Mass Index) by 12/31/2008. Reaching my goal means I never have to have that conversation with my doctor again and I will avoid the need to go on blood pressure medication. I want to live as long as possible and enjoy my retirement to the fullest.

> **Quick Tip**
> Use this website to calculate your current and target BMI:
> http://www.cdc.gov/healthyweight/assessing/index.html

2. *Decide how much you are willing to "pay." What sacrifices are you willing to make consistently for the next 30 days?*

   a. "I will work out for a minimum of 30 minutes on Monday through Saturday for the next 30 days."
   b. "I will limit myself to 1 'treat day' per week for the next 30 days."
   c. "I will trade chips and fries for fruit and vegetables in my meals for the next 30 days."

3. *Do a sanity check:*

   a. Does #2 align with #1? In other words, is what you are willing to pay enough to get you to your goal?

      Yes, I can lose 6 pounds a month if I follow through on the sacrifices planned in step 2 and keep my average calorie count to 1,500 per day (or move more).

   b. Is it something you can <u>reasonably</u> accomplish in the next 30 days? Do you have some "grace" built into your plan?

      Yes! I am not asking too much too soon. Rather than expecting myself to never eat an unhealthy meal, I have committed to cut back but not cut out completely. Having my built in "treat day" to look forward to will help me avoid feeling deprived.

      *Important: If the answer to either of these questions is <u>no</u>, go back and revise your goal!*

4. *Decide how you will reward yourself when you achieve your goal.* Make sure your reward does not conflict with your goal meaning neither rewards or punishments should have anything to do with food or exercise. Additionally, **decide on the penalty if**

**you do not reach it**. Attaching good and negative consequences increases your chances of success.

> If I reach my goal I will: Treat myself to a Swedish massage.

> If I do not reach my goal I will: Forfeit the massage.

---

**Quick Tip**

A blank goal setting worksheet and behavioral contact has been included in the back of this book to help you develop your own plan. You will need to select an accountability partner that is strong enough to hold your feet to the fire (in most instances this means someone outside of your household), yet sensitive enough to provide a word of support and encouragement when needed.

---

I finally had answers and felt good about my goals. They actually seemed realistic and doable.

Food Swap

The next step was identifying the foods that would be included in my meal plan. The guide referenced a substitution plan made up of 5 tiers. To lose weight, I was to focus on swapping the foods I currently ate for similar foods in tiers 1 and 2. Tier 3 was the neutral tier – foods in that category had benefits and hazards. Tier 4 was a slippery slope that should only be enjoyed in small portions and in moderation. Tier 5 was a mine field, the foods tasted great in the short term but you would pay for them dearly in the long term.

Surprise, surprise: many of the foods I currently ate were in tiers 4 and 5. That would further explain why I wasn't getting the results I thought I was working towards. Although I liked the 5-tier system, I realized that I would have to tweak it a bit to make it work for me. I needed to have clear lines of distinction between healthy and not-so-healthy foods, but I also needed to guard against a diet mentality.

*Diet (noun):*

1. Food and drink regularly provided or consumed; habitual nourishment.

2. A regimen of eating and drinking sparingly so as to reduce one's weight.

For once, I wanted to focus on definition #1 rather than definition #2. The reason is simple. Do you remember being told as a kid that you shouldn't or couldn't do something? Do you remember how it made you feel? Back then, someone telling us that we couldn't or shouldn't do something only increased our curiosity and desire to do it. I believe the same is true in adulthood, at least for most of us. The more we tell ourselves what we can't or shouldn't eat, the more we want to eat it…even if it is for our own good.

Instead of making certain foods completely off limits, I decided to break foods into three categories:

1. Everyday foods
2. Sometimes foods
3. Occasional foods

- Everyday foods: I would eat foods from this group every single day because they 1) taste good and 2) are good for me. These foods tend to be relatively low in calories, high in protein, and low in saturated fat, contain low-to-moderate carbs, and consist of little-to-no sugar.
- Sometimes foods: I would eat foods from this group 2-3 times a week (in modest portions). These foods may not be as healthy as everyday foods, but they aren't junk food either. They are generally slightly higher in calories, fats or carbs than my every day foods. Sometimes foods are great because they allow a little variety throughout the week so that I don't have to eat perfectly at every single meal.

- Occasional foods: I would eat foods from this group occasionally (usually once or twice a week) because they provide significantly less nutritional value than every day and sometimes foods. Yep, you guessed it; this category includes foods that are high in calories, saturated fat, carbs, and/or sugar. Processed foods (anything that is not in its original natural state) also fall in this group.

---

**Quick Tip**

Frying automatically drops even the best, most nutritious foods into the occasional category!

---

*Examples of my Everyday foods:*

- Protein shakes
- Vegetables
- Grilled or baked skinless chicken breast
- Grilled or baked fish
- Ground lean turkey (90% lean or better)
- Turkey breast (not deli meat)
- Natural peanut butter
- Almond milk
- Water
- Green tea with stevia
- Hard-boiled Eggs
- Egg whites
- Sweet potato
- Fruit
- Whole grain bread (no high fructose corn syrup)

My everyday food list provides a boatload of health benefits and virtually no draw backs. Foods on the list have very simple, easy-to-read labels because they are whole foods ingredients. While I don't want to go overboard here, I could eat more of these items (especially green veggies) without gaining fat.

*Examples of my Sometimes foods:*

- Brown and wild rice
- Whole grain pasta
- White baked potato
- Lean ground beef (90% or better)
- Lean steak (round, top sirloin)
- Whole wheat crust pizza with 2% cheese and turkey pepperoni
- Turkey bacon
- Canadian bacon
- Canned low-sodium tuna or chicken breast (in water, not oil)
- Shrimp
- Canned low-sodium soup

The foods in my sometimes list are moderately healthy. They have nutritional benefits but may also have some drawbacks (for example, higher in carbs, sugars, or sodium). While the calorie content may not be that much higher than some everyday foods, if eaten too frequently, the fat/carb/sugar content may create a thicker waistline.

*Examples of my Occasional foods:*

- Anything fried
- Fatty ground beef (anything under 90% lean)
- Deli meat, bacon, and sausage (because it's processed)
- Soda, fruit juices, and sweet tea (high in sugar)
- Cookies, candy, cake, ice cream (high in just about everything)
- White pasta (high in processed carbs)
- Sugared cereal (high sugar/carbs, processed)
- Chips, movie theatre popcorn

- Pizza

All of the items on my occasional list are relatively higher in calories, saturated fat, carbs and/or sugars. Since they provide significantly less nutritional value, I would generally limit these items to my treat day and special occasions. They wouldn't be off limits; I would just set boundaries to keep me on track. And because I allowed a little wiggle room, I wouldn't feel deprived. It was so important that I avoid that feeling of deprivation because in the past, that feeling is what derailed my weight loss efforts.

I think I'm happy. I have clear goals and food options that didn't feel overly restrictive.

Now, I needed to figure out how I would translate all of this into a plan that I could execute daily and be guaranteed that I would see results. The approach outlined in the guide seemed solid, but something told me it was easier said than done.

Reflection Points

1. How many calories would you need to target per day to lose 1 pound of fat per week? 2 per week?
2. How much are you willing to pay and for how long in order to reach your goals?
3. What definition of diet have you been using? Has that been helping or hurting you?
4. What is your BMI? Is that okay?

# Chapter 10 – I Knew It Wouldn't Be Easy

> *"All good is hard. All evil is easy. Dying, losing, cheating, and mediocrity is easy. Stay away from easy."*
> ~Scott Alexander

"5 times a day? Who in the world eats 5 times a day?" I thought. The guide and my research touted eating smaller, healthier meals 5-6 times a day as a surefire way to promote weight loss. Purportedly, eating more frequently would help stave off hunger, reducing the risk that I would overeat and boost my metabolism. But was it doable with my crazy schedule?

Extreme Makeover

To follow the schedule and stay within my calorie range, each day would need to look something like this:

| Meal | Timeframe | Calorie Target |
|------|-----------|----------------|
| Breakfast | 7:30 AM – 8:00 AM | 300 |
| Snack 1 | 10:30 AM – 11:00 AM | 150 |
| Lunch | 1:00 PM – 1:30 PM | 450 |
| Snack 2 | 4:00 PM – 4:30 PM | 150 |
| Dinner | 7:00 PM – 7:30 PM | 450 |

**Total** ...................................................................**1,500**

The key to making this approach work was to eat within an hour of waking up and every 2-3 hours thereafter. Breakfast was the most important meal of the day and dinner would have to wrap up at least 3 hours prior to going to bed. Putting an end to eating early in the evening would supposedly put my body into "fat burning mode" all night, priming my body for fat loss. It all sounded good in theory, but I had serious doubts about my ability to pull this one off. As I continued to read, I felt the tension mounting. This was going to be harder than I thought, much harder than I thought.

I had 3 basic problems with this philosophy:

- Going to 5 meals a day sounded like a lot of work. Between my 9-5 that wasn't *really* 9-5 and grad school, more work was the *last thing* I needed.
- I had a storied history with "the most important meal of the day" i.e. breakfast.
- I typically went to bed by 10:30 PM, which meant I would need to eat dinner by 7:30 PM. This rarely happened.

I decided to undergo this lifestyle change in one of the busiest seasons of my life. I was clocking 50-60 hours a week at work and dedicating 20+ hours to school. Having recently added 50 minutes of exercise to the list, I was already feeling overwhelmed. How could I possibly add something else? I hated the thought of having to do more. Even superwoman had her limits.

<u>Mind Over Matter</u>

Trying hard not to over-react, I began thinking it through. Breakfast would be fairly easy. I just needed to get up a little earlier and eat before leaving for work. I could handle that. It was the time between breakfast and dinner that was a problem. My research warned of the evils of snack machines and fast food joints. It was highly recommended that I pack my lunch and snacks to control portions and my calorie intake. Made perfect sense; my concern was the amount of planning that would require. I would have to plan my meals for the week in advance, go shopping, and then prepare and cook the meals. No more winging it. I would actually need to have a plan for how I managed my diet just like I had a plan for managing my money. Ugh. I enjoyed having an area of my life that I didn't have to plan. I often ate breakfast, lunch, and sometimes dinner out simply because of the convenience it offered. I didn't have to think. I just did whatever felt good and was convenient to avoid adding another item to my to-do list. I was willing to pay the price for good health; I just needed a way to balance nutrition and convenience. Was that even possible?

Then I had an epiphany. Who said I couldn't eat out *and* eat healthy? If I could take having to prepare lunch off of my to-do list and just focus on bringing some easy-to-prep snacks, that would relieve a great deal of pressure. As I explored the idea, a huge weight was lifted off of my shoulder. I could breathe again. That would make things manageable. But could I really pull it off? There wasn't a lot of support for the idea of losing weight while eating out and for good reason. There seemed to be connection with Americans' fascination with eating out and their growing waistlines.

*Fast Facts about Americans and Eating Out:*

- 69% of adults age 20 (and over) years are overweight or obese and...
- Americans spend about 46% of their food budget on food prepared away from home and eat 32% of their calories from restaurant or takeout foods.[14]
- One in every four restaurant meals is ordered from a vehicle. Foods ordered most often are hamburgers (37%), sandwiches (15%), pizza (9%) and Mexican food (6%) and...[15]
- People consume 50% more calories, fat and sodium when they eat out than when they cook at home.[16]

It was easy to see how eating out could completely derail your weight loss efforts. Back then, there weren't as many options as there are today. Thanks to pressure from media, legislation, and an increasingly more health conscious society, many restaurants and fast food chains have lighter fare and post the calorie counts of each item.

Still, making the right decision is not a cake walk. It's not easy to skip past the fried chicken tenders, seafood dish that is drowning in creamy sauce and the tasty Italian and order grilled chicken with veggies. No bones about it, it would require discipline to make the choice I knew I should make rather than the one I wanted to make. This would be yet another big adjustment. I would have to re-program myself. I would have to think and act differently than I ever had before and that would not be easy. It was downright scary. But there was hope.

Eight years prior, a man by the name of Jared Fogle received national attention for his "Subway diet".[17] Fogle had become obese by eating junk food and not exercising, but lost a significant amount of weight by eating at Subway. His secret? He made healthier sub selections, ate smaller portions, and cut back on his use of fattening condiments such as mayonnaise. Here was a man who was in the same situation I was and found a way out. He struggled with the same demons, yet found a way to look past the meatball, steak and cheese, and tuna subs and focus on the healthier oven roasted chicken, turkey breast, and club sandwiches. I felt like Jared was on to something. I didn't know him or the depths of his story, but maybe if I could mirror his approach to eating out, I could enjoy similar success? I decided that I was willing to take the risk.

I just couldn't see myself going the rest of my life without periods of time that I would be eating out a lot. My life would include business trips, vacations, and stretches of time where I just didn't have the time or energy to prep and cook a meal at home. I had to learn how to be successful regardless of circumstance. I had to learn how to make better choices. I had to learn how to be more disciplined. I was after something more than a perfect performance; I was on a quest to become a stronger person.

The first step was to come up with a strategy for eating out, just like Jared had. Then I would be willing to try, fail, and learn from my mistakes. I had to allow myself to be human because…I am. I knew I wouldn't always get it right, but I was working on convincing myself that it was okay because I wasn't perfect. With a plan, I could make progress and that's what I was really after. With that the brainstorming began. After hours of research and soul-searching, I came up with a simple, fool-proof strategy that anyone can implement. Anyone includes you.

> *"Setting a goal is not the main thing. It is deciding how you will go about achieving it and staying with that plan."*
> *~Tom Landry*

## TAM'S TIPS FOR EATING OUT

*Strategy #1: Look up the calorie information before ordering to identify healthier selections.*

This was a tip I picked up in my online research. Although eating out was often discouraged, some of the sites recognized that there would be times that it was unavoidable and offered suggestions on how to navigate. The key seemed to be "look before you leap." By taking the time to think very carefully about the results before doing something, I would increase the likelihood that I made the choice that aligned with my goals. I was learning that every decision I made had consequences and it would be wise of me to consider those consequences before making a decision. That was so contrary to how I was used to living – at least from a health standpoint – but it made perfect sense. I had been focusing on the pleasure of eating what I wanted and not considering the pain that would come from it down the road. That was about to change.

I committed to myself that I wouldn't just use Google to find information for research papers or explore travel destinations. I would now use Google to track down the nutritional information on my restaurant of choice so that I could make an informed decision. As I typed in "nutritional information McDonalds" and began navigating around the McDonald's website, I was horrified by what I saw.

McDonald's

| Item | Calories |
|---|---|
| Quarter Pounder with Cheese | 520 |
| Medium Fries | 380 |
| Medium Coke | 200 |
| **Total**.................................................... | **1,100** |

Even if I called myself being "good" at Chick-fil-a, it wasn't much better.

| Item | Calories |
|---|---|
| Cobb Salad | 430 |
| Ranch Dressing | 280 |
| Medium Sweet Tea | 130 |
| **Total**.................................................... | **840** |

My typical meal at Applebee's was a complete disaster!

| Item | Calories |
|---|---|
| ½ Mozzarella Sticks Appetizer | 465 |
| Riblets Basket | 1230 |
| Strawberry Lemonade (2) | 300 |
| **Total**.................................................... | **1,995** |

And Olive Garden was even worse than Applebee's!

| Item | Calories |
|---|---|
| Garden Fresh Salad (2 servings) | 300 |
| Breadsticks (2) | 280 |
| Tour of Italy | 1450 |
| Sprite (2) | 200 |
| **Total**.................................................... | **2,230** |

No wonder I wasn't getting anywhere! Just one of these meals represented anywhere from 55% to 149% of my calorie target for an entire day! Don't get me wrong, I didn't fool myself into thinking these meals were actually healthy, but I had no idea *how unhealthy* they really were. It was easy to think "this one meal won't hurt; I've been good all week." But after seeing how quickly my hard work in my home gym could disappear, doing my research beforehand would be a no-brainer.

---

**Quick Tip**

Apps like *My Fitness Pal* and *Lose It!* can help you quickly and easily track your daily calorie count on your smartphone. Their databases include hundreds of thousands of foods including items at your favorite restaurant. These tools can also help you set reasonable daily calorie targets. Just be aware that the numbers are only estimates; you may need to make adjustments.

---

*Strategy #2: When nutritional information is not available, look for signs in the dish description.*

One of the things that surprised me in my nutritional information research was that there was only a 260 calorie difference between a salad and a burger and fries! As a matter-of-fact, if I simply swapped the Quarter Pounder with a regular cheeseburger, there would only be 40 calories difference between the two. How could this be? It was becoming clear to me that what I thought was the better choice, wasn't always. I could easily think I was doing the right thing, only to find out later that I was better off having what I really wanted! Amazing.

In addition to that, my research taught me that there are some buzz words to watch for in the dish description that would help me avoid high-fat and consequently high-calorie foods at some of my favorite restaurants.

I would need to avoid:

- A La Crème
- Alfredo

- Au Gratin
- Breaded Or Batter-Dipped
- Buttery
- Cheese Sauce or Cheesy
- Creamed or Creamy
- Crisp, Pan Fried, or Fried
- Hollandaise
- Parmesan
- Sauced
- Sautéed
- Smothered
- Stuffed
- Sweet and Sour
- Whipped

And instead choose:

- Baked
- Blackened
- Broiled
- Grilled
- Healthier
- Heart-healthy
- Light
- Low-fat
- Skinny
- Steamed

*Strategy #3: Avoid portion distortion.*

Up until this point, I ate whatever was on my plate. Having grown up hearing about the starving kids in Africa and how fortunate I was to have food to eat, I was conditioned to think that it was my duty, my responsibility, to clean my plate. It turns out that I'm not the only one that thinks that way. This is a big problem because often what is on our plate is way more than what is needed to maintain a healthy weight. It has now come to light that "portion distortion" is a big contributor to the mess we have on our hands in the good old US of A.

Consider these fast facts about portion sizes:

- 20 years ago, a normal portion fast food cheeseburger was 333 calories, today it is 590 calories because these days…[18]
- Restaurant portion sizes may equal to two or three of the standard servings recommended by US Department of Agriculture. And, to add insult to injury…[19]
- Growing portion sizes at restaurants are changing what Americans think of as a "normal" portion at home too.[19] The bottom line: We have been conditioned to overeat!

The US Department of Health and Human Services makes this distinction[20] between portions and serving sizes:

- A *portion* is the amount of food that you choose to eat for a meal or snack. It can be big or small—you decide.
- A *serving* is a measured amount of food or drink, such as one slice of bread or one cup (eight ounces) of milk.

The problem is many foods that are served as a single portion actually contain multiple servings! When we purchase foods in the store, we get a better feel for this by looking at the Nutrition Facts label (which I wasn't used to doing but planned to start). That label tells us the number of servings per package and how many calories are in each serving. After doing some quick math, we can determine if that item is a wise choice. But when you are sitting at a restaurant, you don't have the benefit of a nutrition label. You tend to eat what is served or stop when you get full (even this requires self-control).

If I was going to be successful at losing weight while eating out, I was going to have to be more cognizant of how much I was eating. I could use tricks like ordering from the kid's menu, splitting an entrée with a friend, or asking for a "to-go" box at the onset but again that would require a higher level of discipline than I was used to exercising. Most of all, I needed to re-train myself on what an appropriate portion looked like when eating out or at home. It was time to hit the reset button.

The USDA recommends taking the following steps to get started eating smaller portions[22]:

- Figure out how big your portions really are:
  - Measure how much the bowls, glasses, cups, and plates you usually use hold. Pour your breakfast cereal into your regular bowl. Then, pour it into a measuring cup. How many cups of cereal do you eat each day?

- Measure a fixed amount of some foods and drinks to see what they look like in your glasses and plates. For example, measure 1 cup of juice to see what 1 cup of liquid looks like in your favorite glass.
  - To see what 1 cup, ½ cup, or 1 ounce of some different foods looks like, visit the food gallery at ChooseMyPlate.gov and find some of the foods you eat in each group.
  - Prepare, serve, and eat smaller portions of food. Start by portioning out small amounts to eat and drink. Only go back for more if you are still hungry.

- Pay attention to feelings of hunger. Stop eating when you are satisfied, not full. If there is still food on your plate or on the table, put it away (or throw it out). Repeat the phrase "a moment on the lips, a year on the hips" as you do this.

- A simple trick to help you eat less is to use a smaller plate, bowl, or glass. One cup of food on a small plate looks like more than the same cup of food on a large plate.

- It is important to think about portion sizes when eating out. Order a smaller size option, when it's available. Manage larger portions by sharing or taking home part of your meal. Check out the "When Eating Out, Make Better Choices" page on the ChooseMyPlate.gov website for tips to help you eat only the amount you need when eating out.

- If you tend to overeat, be aware of the time of day, place, and your mood while eating so you can better control the amount you eat. Some people overeat when stressed or upset. Try walking instead of eating, or snack on a healthier option. For example, instead of eating a bag of chips, crunch on some celery, or instead of eating a bowl of ice cream, enjoy a low-fat yogurt with fresh blueberries. Making healthier choices is better for your weight and can also help you feel better.

---

**Quick Tip**

When cooking at home, use a kitchen scale to more accurately measure how many ounces of food you are eating.

---

*Strategy #4: Dodge dish derailers.*

The discovery that the ranch dressing at Chick-fil-a was a whopping 280 calories gave me a clue that it was easy to turn a healthy meal into an unhealthy one in a matter of seconds.

Consider the average number of calories in some of our favorite toppings, condiments, and sauces:

- 3 squirts of ketchup – 50 calories
- 1 tablespoon of butter – 100 calories
- 1 tablespoon of strawberry jam – 50 calories
- 2 tablespoons of peanut butter – 190 calories
- ½ cup maple syrup – 400 calories
- 2 tbsp. barbecue sauce – 50 calories
- 1 tbsp. mayonnaise – 90 calories
- 3 tbsp. tartar sauce – 120 calories
- 1/4 cup teriyaki sauce – 60 calories
- 2 tbsp. sour cream and 2 tsp. butter – 120 calories
- 3 tbsp. cheese sauce – 300 calories

- ¼ cup of Alfredo sauce – 120 calories
- 1 cup of gravy – 120 calories

Yikes! I was shocked by how an "innocent" dish like grilled chicken could move from entrée to dessert-like when I dipped it into just a few tablespoons of sugary barbeque sauce. Then by how adding a dab of mayonnaise on my sandwich instantly boosted my calorie count by 90 and fat content by 10g. Perhaps the biggest shocker, my seemingly healthy side of broccoli spears can easily become a diet derailer just by adding 3 tablespoons of cheese sauce. This was absolute madness! I couldn't believe what I was reading.

Unfortunately, salad dressings weren't the only guilty parties in a typical salad.

Consider this:

- 2 tablespoons of bacon bits – 50 calories
- 10 garlic croutons – 100 calories
- 1 hardboiled egg – 80 calories
- 1/8 cup of craisins – 50 calories
- ½ cup crumbled feta cheese – 90 calories
- 2 tablespoons of Blue Cheese dressing – 150 calories
- 2 tablespoons of Ranch dressing – 150 calories
- 2 tablespoons of Thousand Island dressing – 120 calories
- 2 tablespoons of French dressing – 140 calories
- 2 tablespoons of cream cheese – 150 calories

It wasn't that these items were inherently bad; the danger was in the fact that I was eating these foods unconsciously. I never considered the quality or quantity of condiments, sauces, or toppings I consumed when I thought about how "good" I had been doing with my eating habits. I only thought about the "big stuff" like whether or not I ordered dessert. I had been acting as if these things did not contribute any significant calories to my diet. Bad move.

Armed with my newfound knowledge, I was able to put together a list of guilt-free condiments and toppings:

- Yellow mustard* – 0 calories
- Hot sauce* – 0 calories
- Horseradish* – 0 calories
- Lemon juice – 0 calories
- 1 tbsp. tomato based salsa – 5 calories
- ¼ cup low fat plain yogurt mixed with mustard (replacement for mayo) - 35 calories
- 1 tbsp. light barbeque sauce – 10 calories
- 1 tbsp. reduced sodium soy sauce – 15 calories
- ½ cup canned tomato sauce – 40 calories
- 1 tbsp. balsamic vinegar – 15 calories
- 2 tbsp. fat-free salad dressing (watch sugar content, aim for <5g) – 25 – 50 calories

*Use caution, not all versions are zero calories*

Changing the type of condiments, sauces and toppings I used would need to be a big part of my weight loss strategy.

The Trouble with Breakfast

Breakfast was (and still is) my favorite meal of the day, probably because of the fond childhood memories. I rarely ate breakfast during the school year, but during the summer when I visited my granddad and aunties in "the country," breakfast was the meal I lived for! Bacon, biscuits, and fried potatoes, yum! Something about that combination of food made me smile. Whenever I heard the clamoring of those cast iron pans I knew something good was about to happen. When breakfast was done, we would all gather around the table as a family and eat. You hardly heard a word because everyone was so busy enjoying the food. Those were good times.

Throughout high school, college, and young adulthood, my morning ritual remained the same. As a teenager, I always slept until the last possible minute which sometimes meant that I missed the bus – preparing and eating breakfast would just make me later – no thanks. In college, no way I was getting up to go to the dining hall before 8:00 AM class. I would just get lunch afterwards. By the time I got my first real job, breakfast wasn't even something I thought about. Rarely was I hungry until just a bit before lunch time.

At some point, I started to eat breakfast again. Unfortunately, it wasn't a healthy one. Almost every morning, a few co-workers and I would head down to the cafeteria and nutrition was the last thing on our minds. I bypassed the cereal, fruit, and yogurt and headed straight for the grill. That's where all of the magic happened! Bacon and cheese on a buttered croissant. A Belgian waffle or pancake almost the size of a standard dinner plate with two sides of syrup. On occasion, I would call myself being "good" and pick up a large blueberry muffin and add a pat of butter. To wash it all down, I would pick up a 20 oz. bottle of orange juice or Lipton Green tea. I didn't realize it at the time, but this one meal often caused the entire day to spiral out of control. At lunch and dinner I sought to replicate the high from breakfast. Like a druggie, I was always looking for my next fix. Now, I would get my high another way.

I learned that eating a healthy breakfast, like exercise, would improve my quality of life, not just my waistline. A balanced breakfast would provide a boost of energy and help me think more clearly; two things I desperately needed to balance my career and school workload. As much as I enjoyed the taste of my comfort food breakfast, it wasn't providing any added benefits. I often felt sluggish after eating it rather than being energized.

Nutritionists and dieticians also cited an added benefit: starting my day with a healthy breakfast would increase the chances that I would make healthy eating choices *throughout the entire day* and as a result, I could end up eating fewer total calories. A study at the University of Texas at El Paso found that 400 calories consumed earlier in the day is more filling than if the same 400 calories were eaten later on, lessening overall calorie consumption. I needed all the help I could get and was willing to give it a try.

Now if I could only jump that last hurdle – dinner time.

<u>The Dinner Time Dilemma</u>

According to my handy dandy nutrition guide, eating late at night was a no-no. I needed to shut it down by 7:30 PM to ensure my body was in "fat burning mode" by the time I went to bed at 10:30 PM. The difficulty with that was that my childhood dream of finding a job that paid well without working long hours wasn't yet reality. It wasn't uncommon for me to leave the office around 7:00 PM. By the time I got home and settled, it was 7:30 PM – 8:00 PM. I was worried. With my current schedule, there was no way I would consistently be in compliance with the 3-hour rule. Did this mean that my 6-pound-a-month goal was in jeopardy?

Interestingly enough there were mixed reviews on the 3-hour rule online. Some agreed with the fat burning mode viewpoint, but there seemed to be more that contended that there was no proof that the very act of eating before bed led to weight gain; a calorie was still a calorie regardless of when it was eaten.

After evaluating my own habits, I found that I had my own personal reasons to push up my dinner time. For me, eating late at night generally meant a poor food choice. I was tired and hungry (because I had waited too late and not planned appropriately) and was likely to grab what was convenient, not what was nutritious. Trying to stick as closely as possible to the 3-hour rule would force me to leave work at a more reasonable time and either prepare my meals in advance or ensure that I had something quick and healthy to prepare. It was going to be a challenge but maybe this was God's way of forcing me to set boundaries. Boundaries I needed to set long ago.

<u>Sugar High</u>

I had made a lot of progress sorting out my issues with meal planning, but there was something bothering me. I had gotten into a habit of eating something sweet immediately after dinner. It became somewhat of a ritual, a happy ending to my day. I cringed at the thought of looking up the nutritional information on some of my favorite treats because I figured the results wouldn't be flattering. Boy was I right about that!

- Little Debbie Swiss Cake rolls – 270 calories, 26 grams of sugar
- Butterfinger bar – 270 calories, 28 grams of sugar
- Mrs. Smith's Apple Pie singles with ½ cup of French vanilla ice cream – 400 calories, 23 grams of sugar
- 3 Pillsbury chocolate chip cookies – 390 calories, 33 grams of sugar
- 1 cup Breyers Cookies and Cream Ice Cream – 280 calories, 30 grams of sugar
- 3 Sweet 16 white powdered donuts – 230 calories, 14 grams of sugar

For the first time, I started to pay attention to the sugar totals. The numbers seemed high but I had trouble relating to them in grams. I began to search for a way that I could convert the grams into something meaningful. Here's what I found:

**4 grams of sugar = 1 teaspoon**

Now it was time to do the math:

- Little Debbie Swiss Cake rolls – 7 teaspoons of sugar
- Butterfinger bar – 7 teaspoons of sugar
- Mrs. Smith's Apple Pie singles with ½ cup of French vanilla ice cream– 6 teaspoons of sugar
- 3 Pillsbury chocolate chip cookies – 8 teaspoons of sugar
- 1 cup Breyers Cookies and Cream Ice Cream – 8 teaspoons of sugar
- 3 Sweet 16 white powdered donuts – 4 teaspoons of sugar

I couldn't believe that I was regularly eating the equivalent of 4-8 teaspoons of sugar after every dinner meal! No wonder I was struggling to even maintain my weight. I found a little comfort in the fact that my research indicated that I wasn't the only one. America had a sugar problem that continued to worsen with every passing year. Food manufacturers were putting out fat-free and low-fat foods, in response to customer demand for healthier options, but added sugar to make up for the difference in taste. The result? Americans were becoming sugar fiends.

---

### Did You Know?

Experiments in animals and humans show that, for some people, the same reward and pleasure centers of the brain that are triggered by addictive drugs like cocaine and heroin are also activated by food, especially foods rich in sugar, fat, and salt.[23]

The American Public Health Administration recommends that the average adult consume no more than 40 grams per day. The majority of sugars consumed should be "natural sugars" (ex. fruits) vs. "added sugars" (ex. Table sugar, corn syrup).

What are the effects of sugar? Sugar increases insulin levels temporarily. A short while later, you "crash" and are left feeling tired and hungry. The worst part is you will crave more sugar! It's a vicious cycle.

---

According to a recent Forbes article,[24] Americans consume about:

- 3 pounds of sugar each week
- 130 pounds of sugar per year
- A whopping 3,550 pounds of sugar in a lifetime, the equivalent of 1,767,900 Skittles!

As a country, we were out of control and I was one of the ring leaders. I learned that not only were the candies, cakes, cookies, and pies a problem, but also the sodas and fruit drinks that I drank regularly. Both were laden with sugar and high in calories (150 calories or more for one 12 oz. can) and the more I drank them, the more I fueled my sugar cravings. It became clear that I needed to stop eating and drinking so much sugar. But could I stop cold turkey?

## The Weaning Period

Like any addict, I worried about my ability to quit just like that. I decided that I would cut back drastically but still allow myself to be human. I would create a guilt-free plan that ensured I would reach my goals without going into "withdrawal."

The game plan:

- A limit of one 12 oz. canned soda or fruit juice per day.
- A minimum intake of 8 glasses (64 oz. of water per day).
- I could have one low-calorie dessert per day, typically a 100-calorie Little Debbie Pinwheel or 150-calorie Pet Ice Cream Sandwich.
- I would aim to meet the Center for Disease Control recommendation[25] of 2 cups of fruit per day, which would help reduce my cravings.

This meant I needed to go back to my Goal Setting Worksheet and make some changes to item #2.

*Decide how much you are willing to "pay." What sacrifices are you willing to make consistently for the next 30 days?*

    a. "I will workout for a minimum of 30 minutes on Monday through Saturday for the next 30 days."
    b. "I will limit myself to 1 'treat day' per week for the next 30 days."
    c. "I will trade chips and fries for fruit and vegetables in my meals for the next 30 days."
    **d. "I will only drink 1 soda per day for the next 30 days."**
    **e. "I will limit myself to one treat of 150 calories or less per day for the next 30 days."**

*Note: I followed this plan for about 30 days and eventually I found that I didn't need the sugar high as often – at least not from processed foods. The naturally occurring sugar in fruit was giving me a sufficient sweet fix and I was able to make soda and the Little Debbie's all an occasional indulgence. I am a witness, if you stick with it long enough, your taste buds can and do change!*

<u>Tying Up Loose Ends</u>

After sorting through my eating dilemma, I realized that something was still missing. I had basic guidelines for how I would eat, but I knew I had not gotten specific enough. What exactly would I eat for breakfast, lunch, and dinner? What about snacks? How would I ensure all of these meals would be within the range of calories that I needed? There was still way too much ambiguity for my taste. I needed to make it easy for me to succeed rather than make it easy for me to fail.

I decided I would create my own "menu" comprised mostly of my everyday foods. I would create combinations that aligned with my calorie targets and then pick and choose which combo would be a part of my plan for that week. I would rotate my selections regularly to avoid getting bored and was constantly on the hunt for new recipes. I realized from past experience that boredom was the enemy. I had to avoid it at all costs!

## MY MENU

Ideally, each mini-meal should include lean or low-fat protein, fiber, a little healthy fat, and at least one fruit or veggie.

*Breakfast:*

- A protein shake (with fiber and a small amount of polyunsaturated and/or monounsaturated fat)
- A smoothie with low-fat yogurt and fruit
- Egg whites, a slice of whole wheat toast, half a grapefruit
- A slice of whole wheat toast with 1 tbsp. peanut butter and a small banana
- Breakfast parfait with low fat yogurt, 1/2-cup fresh chopped fruit and 1/3-cup low-fat granola, low sugar granola.
- An apple with a piece of low-fat cheese
- 2 slices of turkey bacon or Canadian bacon, egg whites and ½ a slice of cheese

*Lunch:*

- Hibachi chicken or salmon with veggies and green onion soup (no rice or noodles)
- Mexican chicken burrito bowl with rice, lettuce, and tomato salsa
- Fast food grilled chicken sandwich with side salad and ½ packet of reduced fat dressing
- Fast food grilled chicken salad and ½ - ¾ packet of reduced fat dressing
- Grilled Salmon Salad with Balsamic Vinaigrette dressing

*Dinner:*

- Roasted/grilled, broiled/baked chicken and brown rice with steamed string beans
- Salmon and stir fried veggies
- Grilled chicken topped with salsa and a side of asparagus
- Turkey burger with 2% cheese on wheat, sweet potato
- Vegetable soup with grilled 2% cheese sandwich
- Turkey spaghetti with whole wheat noodles and low fat cheese and a side salad
- Grilled chicken with a hint of light BBQ sauce, lima beans, and corn

---

**Quick Tip: My Favorite Recipe Websites**

SparkPeople.com

LiveBetterAmerica.com

CookingLight.com

Webmd.com

---

The Blessing of Boundaries

After talking myself off of the emotional ledge a few times, I felt good about the work I had done. Though aggravating initially, I found that taking the time to develop a structured plan actually *reduced* my stress levels.

We rarely think of it this way but I've come to realize that boundaries create freedom. Think about it. When you have proper boundaries, you have freedom from worry. Freedom from the fear of negative consequences. Freedom from guilt.

For the first time, I felt empowered to successfully navigate the journey ahead. I knew what I needed to do and how I needed to do it. It wasn't going to be easy, but nothing worth having is. Best of all, this time, I honestly believed I could do it and that made all the difference.

---

**Quick Tip**

As long as your meals are well-distributed through the day, and you never go more than 4-5 hours without food, you can reach your weight loss goals with three, four, five, or six meals a day. Do what works for you!

---

Reflection Points

1. Google the nutrition information for some of your favorite indulgences. Given your daily calorie target, how often can you afford to indulge in this way?
2. What adjustments do you need to make in your eating habits in order to lose the weight and keep it off?
3. How close are you to the recommended 40 grams of sugar or less per day?

14. Ksre.ksu.edu, 2007

15. Ksre.ksu.edu, 2007

16. USAtoday30.usatoday.com, 2004

17. Wikipedia.com, n.d.

18. Nhlbi.nih.gov, 2013

19. Ksre.ksu.edu, 2007

20. Nhlbi.nih.gov, 2013

21. Nhlbi.nih.gov, 2013

22. Choosemyplate.gov, 2013

23. Webmd.com, 2013

24. Forbes.com, 2012

25. CDC.gov, 2013

# Chapter 11 -The Unexpected

"Are you losing weight?" my mom said as I settled into the passenger seat of her car. It was now March of 2008. I was almost three months into my journey and nearly two months into changing my eating *and* exercise habits. "I might have lost a few pounds" I said sheepishly. Sensing my discomfort, mom let it go and we went about our day. Unfortunately, the conversation continued in my mind.

Ignorant Bliss

I wasn't sure how many pounds I had lost. This time around I was trying not to focus so much on the scale. In the past, I had weighed myself daily and sometimes several times a day hoping for some glimmer of hope that things were moving in the right direction. More often than not, it backfired. My weight fluctuated from day to day and during the day for reasons I didn't then understand. I would walk away from my bathroom ashamed, dejected, and discouraged. I decided that this time, I would focus on doing the right things and leave the results to God. I couldn't always control what showed up on that scale, but I could control whether or not I was doing the right things. As long as I was getting in the exercise and watching my calories like I planned, there was nothing to worry about. I decided that I no longer needed the scale to validate me. I knew I was on the right track and that was such an unbelievable feeling -- one that I could easily get used to.

That wasn't to say that the last few months had been easy. I was proud of myself for getting in workouts daily and following through on my commitment to have just one soda and one treat per day, but I hadn't been flawless. There were a few days I could only get in one of two workouts because my schoolwork demanded my attention. There was more than one occasion where I went over my target calorie count. I tried not be too hard on myself, but as a perfectionist with a less-than-perfect performance, worry set in. The situation I feared had come to pass and I was concerned that it would be my undoing. But somehow I managed to shove those feelings to the back of my mind, hoping they would eventually go away. They did – temporarily - and despite my slip ups, what I was doing was working. My persistence was paying off, so why was I feeling so uneasy?

## The Big Uneasy

I hadn't told my mom or anyone about the details of my last doctor's office visit and only told one or two people about my decision to take control of my health. It wasn't that I couldn't have used their support; Lord knows I could have, but I held back because I was afraid. Afraid of failure and at the same time afraid of success. I had been fearful of the very moment I was now experiencing. The moment when what you are doing is noticeable to others. The moment when your actions are speaking louder than your words. The moment when you are exposed for all the world to see. The moment you stop becoming invisible.

> *"Comfort zones are most often expanded through discomfort."*
> *~Peter McWilliams*

I had been hiding behind my weight for a long time. It was like that layer of fat covered up all of the sadness, guilt, and shame I felt. Sadness because I didn't feel as though I was good enough. Guilt that I had allowed myself to get to this point. Shame because as strong as I claimed to be, I couldn't find the courage to turn this situation around. I felt like a failure and somehow, someway, the weight allowed me to hide that. Being fat was a conduit for burying those emotions. I became a pale figure on a pale background, utterly indistinguishable. As strange as it may seem, there was comfort in that.

When I started my journey, I wasn't very confident in myself. The extra pounds I was carrying around were weighing on my body and my mind. Deep down, I felt unworthy of love. Negative thoughts plagued my mind and reflected in my words, actions, and habits. I walked around with my head down and shoulders slouched. I almost never made eye contact because I believed that the eyes were the windows to the soul, and mine was lost. I wasn't very happy and for the life of me, I didn't know how to change that.

But now things were different. I was starting to taste success and feel better about myself. I could go longer periods of time without taking a break in the workout. I was full of energy. I felt lighter and more alive. I was starting to like who I was again, on the inside as well as the outside. It felt good and eerie at the same time. Losing weight was supposed to be a good thing yet it came with its own set of unexpected problems.

## My Mind is Playing Tricks on Me

One of the benefits of me keeping my journey to myself was that I didn't have to deal with added pressure. Since I was the only person that knew the details of what I was doing, I was the only person I had to be accountable to. Fortunately, I had been holding myself accountable, but having others do it was a whole different ball game. If my mom noticed, soon other people would too. They would be watching what I ate, asking me what I was doing to get results and waiting to see if I would continue to make progress. That was a lot of pressure. A burden I wasn't sure I was prepared to deal with. I felt extremely vulnerable and I never really liked that feeling.

Plus I was terrified that this success could end up being one big set up. That the innocent little compliment that my mom tried to give me would end up biting me in the rear as it had so many times before. Her compliment was confirmation that I was headed for victory and that was a major problem. Instead of continuing to work hard when I tasted triumph, I had a tendency to ease up a little. I would start to think, "Hey, this isn't so bad," and that was a dangerous thought; one that was quickly followed with "I've got this!" and next thing I know I am slacking off and cutting corners. Spend enough time in that mental space and you end up gradually negating all of your hard work until you're right back where you started and you have no idea how you got there. What seemed to be a harmless thought was anything but.

I had felt so confident in my ability to beat this thing once and for all, and now with the asking of one simple question, I was questioning everything. Could this flawed, unworthy, outcast really achieve success? Or would I cave under the pressure and give up on it all? I wanted to believe that I could push past this, but how could I be sure?

I finally had the blueprint I had been looking for. I had proven to myself that following it produced great results. It stood to reason that if I just kept doing what I was doing, I would eventually reach my goal. Simple right? Maybe, but simple is not the same as easy and truth is, I had a thing for easy. Given a choice, I always preferred the path of least resistance. The sure bet. The layup. I liked to win. I hated to lose.

In my mind, even a minor loss was synonymous with being a loser. Whenever I didn't perform perfectly at work, in school, or in a relationship, feelings of failure and inadequacy were sure to follow. Once again, I didn't measure up. I let someone down. Something was missing. I was incomplete. In my desperate attempt to avoid such feelings, I shut myself out from much of the world. I was a prisoner of my own thoughts.

I became a very successful quitter. I was successful because I generally only took high percentage shots. Now that didn't mean that if I took a shot, I thought that I was guaranteed a victory, but rather that I believed I was capable of accomplishing the task. Whenever I doubted my ability, my modus operandi was to abandon ship. I became very good at evading situations that posed a risk to my self-image and psyche.

- I quit track in middle school because I got embarrassed in a practice relay.
- I came very close to changing majors in undergrad because for once, academics didn't come easy.
- I seriously considered giving up on my dream of going to grad school because I didn't get in the first time around.
- After a string of bad relationships, I quit thinking I deserved better and settled for guys that treated me like trash.
- When I did meet a decent guy, I broke up with him at the first sign of difficulty rather than risk him leaving me.
- I quit on my dream of losing weight because I hated feeling like a big old failure every time I messed up.

Fear was setting in and starting to get the best of me. My thoughts were spiraling out of control. I imagined the worst possible outcome: I'd eventually reach my goal only to gain it all back. I would be the laughing stock of my family, friends, and co-workers. Once and for all, everyone would know how big of a screw up that I was. It was only a matter of time. I tried to put the self-sabotaging thoughts out of my mind, but each time I pushed them away, they only seemed to resurface.

Physically I continued to make progress, but I was mentally and emotionally drained. I now felt as though I had something to prove and that made me work even harder. I added time to my workouts. I forfeited some treat days. I became obsessed with the scale. All appeared to be well on the outside, but on the inside I was in a state of turmoil. It felt like the more driven I was, the more sacrifices I made, the more consistent my behavior, the more I felt that my house of cards would soon come tumbling down. I was hanging on by a thread, trying desperately not to let go.

Weeks passed and suddenly it was my 34th birthday. I began to reflect and remembered that a very important date was just around the corner.

Reflection Points

1. How have you been hiding behind your weight?
2. When it comes to health and fitness, do you tend to let faith or fear rule? How?

# Chapter 12 - The Intervention

"Your position has been eliminated," my manager said. With that, I, the woman who was generally cool, calm and collected, started to tear. She kept talking but I can't really tell you what she said. As I watched her lips move "why is this happening to me?" kept playing over and over in my head. I just couldn't wrap my mind around it. We all knew that something was up because the trip came up out of the blue, but I had no idea that this was the intention of the visit. I felt betrayed.

How Did I Get Here?

It was April of 2004 and just a few months prior, my manager and her boss had been singing my praises at an offsite meeting. Each of us was required to present on several subjects while our teammates and managers evaluated us. Like everyone, I had butterflies, but my experience in *Toastmasters* had prepared me well for this. The feedback served as confirmation. I was commended for my organization and knowledge of the material, strong communication skills, and something they referred to as "presence." Nice.

I was especially happy because the feedback I received that day was a complete 180 from what I heard the first time I presented. Five years prior, I went on my first interview for a training job and the shy, introvert in me was completely thrown by the panel interview. I sweated bullets the entire time and wasn't at all surprised when I didn't get the job. But I had resolved that I would be back. I felt a strong sense, a call if you will, to teach. Although the outward manifestation had not come, I believed I could do it. Finally, I had. I put in necessary work to develop my craft and now I was living my dream. I loved that job and couldn't imagine doing anything else. My spirit was crushed.

## An Olive Branch

Suddenly, it dawned on me that one of my business partners was in the room. I'm sure she was there all the time. I had just been so distracted by the news that I hadn't noticed. After my manager finished her spiel, my business partner put her hand on my shoulder, handed me a tissue and told me not to worry. She was going to find me something. That she did, but it wasn't at all what I expected.

I was offered the same job I had been training people to perform for the last 2 years. While thankful for the opportunity to continue my employment, I couldn't help but feel like I was taking a step back. I had worked really hard to get where I was and it felt like I was finally in the zone. I loved teaching and the thought of no longer doing it made me sick to my stomach. Still, if I didn't take the job, it would only be a few months before my severance would run out. I would have to find something comparable fast or potentially risk losing everything. I didn't know what to do.

> *"I seem to have run in a great circle, and met myself again on the starting line."*
> ~Jeanette Winterson

I had so many questions. Should I take the job to keep a steady paycheck? Or take the severance and look for a job at another bank? Maybe this was an opportunity to start my own training business? The more I thought about each option, the more confused I became. I was deathly afraid of making a mistake that would alter the course of my life forever. I told my business partner thank you and asked her to give me the weekend to think about her offer.

## The Good Life

I decided that I needed the input of wise counsel - my mom, my uncle, and my pastor. My mom allowed me to vent my frustrations and my aspirations then assured me that she would support me either way. My uncle was confident that it was a temporary setback and encouraged me to take the job while continuing to look for another opportunity. My pastor told me that regardless of what decision I made, I could have faith that it would ultimately work out for my good.

I had heard the "all things work together for the good" reference on many occasions but this time it really hit home -- all things – good things and bad things. Up until this point, this was the worst thing that had happened to me, so surely this had to qualify! If it was true that all things worked together for my good, then I didn't need to worry about making a decision that would ruin my life. The path I chose may determine how long it takes me to get from point A to point B, but in any event, I would eventually get there. I had to. Because faith never fails. Understanding this really took the pressure off. I was ready to make a decision without anxiety. I knew what I had to do, but I wasn't looking forward to it.

## Anywhere But Here

I walked into the office on Monday morning and told my business partner that I would take the job. I had peace that it was the right thing to do, but somehow it didn't feel right, if you know what I mean. I felt like I had been held back from advancing to the next grade; like I was in remedial classes because I had failed to meet the minimum standard. What did I do wrong? How did I go from having "presence" to being a has been? I was trying to move forward, but deep down I was bitter over the decision. I didn't think I deserved it. My confidence was shaken. I felt that I had been cheated.

Instead of preparing for and facilitating classes, I would be sitting behind a desk all day staring at a computer. Most of the tasks would be repetitive which in my mind meant less of a challenge. On top of that, all eyes would be on me to see if I could do as well as teach. It was tough for me to find something positive about this situation, but at least I still had a job. There was something in me that said that this wasn't the end. I would be back, better and stronger. I had destiny on my side.

I stayed in the job 9 months, ironically the same timeframe as a normal pregnancy. Like a pregnant woman, I experienced morning sickness daily. I absolutely dreaded my work and the thought of going in made me nauseous. A few times, I considered giving my notice. I wanted to be anywhere but there. I didn't know I would be stuck in the position that long. Maybe I had made a mistake? But somehow, someway I found the strength to keep showing up, relying on my faith to sustain me. Finally there was a break in the dam.

## Daybreak

After 9 months of no's, I finally got a break and landed an assistant manager position in the Sales department. Within 18 months, I was managing my own team. My pastor was right. It did work out for my good in the end.

Being reminded of all of this put my current situation into a new light. In 2004, I had been fearful of the attention that would be on me. I was shaken and insecure. I didn't know if I had the strength to make it. I wanted to stick my tail between my legs and run. But I didn't. I took it day by day and kept going. Eventually I came out on the other side. Maybe my weight loss journey would be similar? If I just stomached the ups and downs, if I didn't quit, if I relied on my faith, I would make it. As I continued to reflect, my fears began to recede and my convictions began to rise. I *have* been here before. I can do this.

## The X Factor

It wasn't my mom's question that was the problem. It was how I responded to the question. A self-sabotaging thought surfaced and I allowed it to fester and grow. I was responsible for my emotional state. No one else. If I was going to come out of this a winner, I was going to have to change my thoughts. It wasn't what others said or did that was most important. It was what I said to myself that mattered and my words originated with my thoughts.

You may not believe in the power of positive thinking, but I cannot emphasize enough how important what you think and say is. I am convinced that what you think is THE determining factor in whether or not you reach your health and fitness goals. It is a very strong statement, but I stand behind it 100%.

"Stinking thinking" is the #1 reason we don't stick to our commitments. Allow me to prove it to you.

Have you ever thought these or similar thoughts?

- "Losing weight is too hard."
- "I am too lazy to lose weight."
- "When I see/smell xyz, I just can't help myself."
- "It's just the way I am. I'm always going to be fat."
- "It's just too much pressure"
- "It runs in the family."
- "I don't have time to exercise."
- "I am too clumsy to exercise"
- "I can't afford to eat healthier."
- "Planning healthy meals takes too much time."
- "Eating healthy is boring."
- "It's taking too long to get results. What I'm doing must not be working."
- "I don't x, y, z, I've got to have something."
- "I just don't have the willpower."
- "I ate something bad this morning...so I might as well enjoy the rest of the day and start again tomorrow (or Monday)!"
- "My boss really made me mad. I need a mental break."
- "The kids are driving me nuts. Eating some XXX will make me feel better."
- "I knew this would happen."
- "See, I told you that you couldn't do it!"

In each of these scenarios, one of two things (or both) is happening:

- We believe that the way we feel or act is a result of someone else's actions or some external event.
- We are playing the victim.

The root of these thoughts is a four letter word: fear. Fear that you are incapable of change. Fear that you are not strong enough. Fear that you are not good enough. Fear that you will fail, or succeed. If you don't put fear in its place, and fast, it can easily get out of control. It's a slippery slope; a domino effect. You start to hear the nagging voices. You entertain the negative thoughts. Your confidence begins to fade. You start to question everything. Your commitment. Your abilities. Your faith. You start to think that this time will be like all the other times. Soon, everyone will know your secret - you never really changed. You had some victories, but you are not a winner. You are an imposter and your cover is about to be blown.

When these thoughts emerge, you have to fight back. And the sooner, the better, because your success depends on it. Still not sure?

Allow me to share one of my favorite quotes. It will connect the dots:

> *"Watch your thoughts, for they become words.*
>
> *Watch your words, for they become actions.*
>
> *Watch your actions, for they become habits.*
>
> *Watch your habits, for they become character.*
>
> *Watch your character, for it becomes your destiny."*
>
> *~Author Unknown*

A quick fill-in-the-blank exercise…

1. What I say out of my mouth, comes from what I am
   _____.
2. What I say will eventually determine what I will _____.
3. If I do something long enough it becomes a _____.
4. And what I do consistently is a reflection of my
   _____.
5. My character, or the kind of person I am on a consistent
   basis, will determine my _____.
6. So ultimately, where I am going to be emotionally, financially,
   physically, etc. 1, 2, 3 or 5 years from now depends on my
   _____.

*Answer Key: 1) thinking, 2) do, 3) habit, 4) character, 5) destiny, 6) thoughts*

## Thought Replacement

We must all drown out the voice of the inner critic that says, "No I can't," and fight back with "yes, I can" messages. But how do we do it?

- Be honest with yourself about what you will and will not do
- Set realistic goals
- Make it easy for you to succeed and hard to fail
- Practice exercising discipline in small things. It adds up.
- Don't make promises to yourself that you are not ready to keep
- Take it one day at a time
- Celebrate your victories (without food)
- Focus on progress and not perfection
- Feed what you want to grow

Again, these things are not easy. Remind yourself to be patient. We tend to believe our personality, attitude, and level of discipline are fixed — that no matter what we do, we won't improve, but this too is faulty thinking. If we keep at it and focus on getting better rather than being perfect, take adversity in stride, and learn to enjoy the journey rather than obsessing over the destination, life and weight loss will be so much more rewarding. But here's the thing: It all starts with what you think. Others believing for you will only carry you so far; you must believe deep down that you have what it takes.

## Mission Possible

No matter how many times you've tried and failed, you have the power to change your life. Whether you want to lose 20, 30, 50, or even 100 pounds, you can do it; if you believe that you can. Yes, it's going to take hard work. Yes, your emotions will be all over the place. Yes, there will be days that you want to quit. Yes, there will be days that you fall short. You may even be frightened that you'll be a success or failure, but it doesn't have to stay that way. Even at the core of your being, you can change.

To change the direction of your life, change the direction of your thoughts.

## Reflection Points

1. What stinking thinking have you bought into?
2. What actions will you take to begin reprogramming your mind?

# Chapter 13 - So This is What Success Smells Like

*"It is a rough road that leads to the heights of greatness."*
*~Lucius Annaeus Seneca*

"Come here!" my friend "Sasha" said as she motioned me over to her desk. She was so emphatic about it that I abandoned my intended route and started walking in her direction. When I got to her desk she said "Girl! Your pants are about to fall off of you!" She immediately started asking around for safety pins and pulled me into a nearby conference room so that she could doctor up my outfit. "I need to find out what you've been doing! The weight is just falling off of you!" she said. "Sasha" knew that I was trying to lose weight but not much else.

The Secret is Out

Even though we were very good friends, I didn't want to jinx myself by talking too much about what I was doing. Talk was cheap and I had been full of cheap stuff before. This time I wanted my results to speak for themselves and finally they were talking!

"Sasha" put a safety pin on both sides of my pants, laughed and said, "That will have to do." We both laughed and talked for a while. I promised to share with her the nuggets I had picked up about the importance of nutrition and with that we concluded that we had better get back to work.

I opened the door to the conference room and it was all eyes on me. Several people in the office were looking in my direction and whispering amongst themselves. I tried just smiling and saying hello as I always did, hoping that they would leave it at that. That didn't happen. "Girl, you're looking good! What are you doing?" one of my co-workers said. I replied, "Just trying to eat right and exercise," and kept it moving. The questions continued. No one could believe it; it couldn't be that simple! I assured them that it was, not realizing how elementary it sounded. I was a little embarrassed by all of the attention, but I didn't doubt myself like I did before. The time I spent in prayer and meditation each morning was working.

I would get similar reactions throughout the day and even in the weeks to come. One of the male security guards even stopped me in the hall to compliment me and ask me about my "secret." I responded with the same eat-right-and-exercise comment as I had before, but the questions persisted. "What do you eat?" "How often do you exercise?" "How long have you been doing it?" As quickly as the questions came, I tried to answer them. It was crazy; I became an office phenomenon overnight.

I still can't explain what happened that day. It started out like any other. I worked out, had breakfast, and ironed my clothes. After I got out of the shower, I got dressed and realized the outfit I planned to wear was way too big. I went back to the closet and pulled out another outfit, but it didn't fit either. I tried outfit after outfit and they were all too big. I grew frustrated and decided "this will have to do!" Thinking I had chosen the lesser of many evils, I rushed out of the door. I didn't realize how baggy my pants were. I had to laugh at the whole situation. I never thought that my clothes falling off would be a side effect of losing weight, but it felt so good.

Shop 'Til I Drop

After all of the attention I received that day, it became clear that I needed to go shopping. I headed to the usual spot, Lane Bryant. I grabbed a few size 14 W pants and headed into the dressing room. I was excited at the prospect of wearing such a small size. Having worn a 24 W at one point and an 18 W the last time I went shopping, it was a big accomplishment. As I slipped on the pants, zipped them and looked in the mirror, I was amazed by what I saw. The 14 W was too big! Thinking it was a fluke, I tried on the remaining pairs of pants. Same result. I didn't know what to do.

As strange as it may seem, I became emotional. I sat on the fitting room bench and began to tear. I was getting the results I wanted all along but somehow I hadn't envisioned this moment. A store that I had shopped at for 8 years, no longer had clothes that fit me. I was traumatized. I sat there, almost paralyzed. I needed clothes and nothing fit. What was I supposed to do?

I wasn't thinking clearly but thankfully I had sense enough to call my girl "Sasha." I explained my situation and in true "Sasha" style she said, "Girl, go to the mall!" With hesitation, I replied, "The mall?" She said, "Girl, yes. The mall!" I hung up with "Sasha," put the clothes on the rack and left the store. But not before heading into the nearby Dress Barn. I tried on a few clothes in their plus sized section with the same outcome. Finally I conceded and headed to the mall.

I'm not sure why I was so resistant to the idea of going the mall. Perhaps it was because it had been so long since I shopped there. After graduating from the Misses section to the Women's department, I just didn't see the point in going. The selection was poor and I felt out of place. But now, I had nowhere else to go. Like it or not, the mall and I were about to be reacquainted.

Based on the experience at Lane Bryant and Dress Barn, I knew there was no point in going to the plus sized section, but I had no idea what size I wore! I decided to grab a variety of sizes and head to the dressing room. After a few trips to the department store floor and back, I finally settled on a size 12. I could even wear a 13/14 juniors in some brands. I was blown away...and completely and totally exhausted! Who knew that losing weight could be such an emotionally trying experience? Still, it was still worth it. I was doing it! I was really doing it!

I needed a whole new wardrobe but I couldn't afford to spend that kind of cash. Thankfully, one of my friends at work "Tasha" noticed my plight and offered to sell me some of her clothes.

"Tasha" had amazing style and I jumped at the opportunity. She had a spare bedroom full of suits, pants and blouses that she was willing to sell and acted as my personal shopper. "Tasha" selected various outfits that she knew would complement my new shape. As I tried them on, I was amazed that we actually wore the same size. "Tasha" and I wore the same size! Pinch me, I must be dreaming!

I wasn't dreaming. Since changing my eating habits, I had lost 50 pounds. Considering the rocky start, I was super proud of myself. I was on track to reach my goal by year end. I just had to keep going.

Model Behavior

It wasn't long before people in the office started treating me differently. I felt eyes peering at me as I took snacks out of my lunch bag. My selections at office potlucks were under scrutiny. When I went out to lunch and came back with a McDonald's bag, I was asked, "What are you doing eating at McDonalds?" It was an interesting change of events, just as I expected. I was on stage. Like it or not, I had become a role model. Others were looking to me to set the example.

I accepted the challenge and began offering to help others reach their goals. Those that followed my advice started seeing results. It felt good to help others. It was the perfect marriage – my teaching abilities and a topic of epic proportions. I was making a difference. Once 100 pounds overweight, I was now an agent of change. What a scary but exhilarating thought. Lives were being changed and I was blessed to be a part of it.

Reflection Points

1. Imagine that you have reached your goal weight. How would that feel?
2. Knowing how difficult it is to lose weight, how would you pay it forward?

# Chapter 14 -  Fearing Fear

The day I had been working for all year was finally here. It was October 17, 2008, and the scale read 164 pounds. I was no longer obese or even overweight. My BMI was below 25. I was at a healthy weight. Words could not express the gratification I felt! All of the hard work over the past 10 months had finally paid off. I did it! I really did it!

What I was most proud of was that in the weeks to follow I didn't relax. I kept working out and eating right even though I had met my goal. I learned a valuable lesson from my relapse in 2006: whatever you do to lose the weight, you have to keep doing to maintain it. I had been working out 6 days a week for 10 months, eating better for 9. It was truly becoming a habit. I wasn't dieting, I was living. Living with a newfound sense of self-control. Living with vitality and energy. Living on purpose. But could I really keep this up during the most wonderful time of the year?

## The Most Wonderful Time of the Year

The six weeks between Thanksgiving and Christmas had long been a favorite of mine. For me and my family, it was a time set aside to celebrate what we are most thankful for. A time to show appreciation for all of the blessings we'd been given. A season of giving, not only of material things, but of ourselves through intentional fellowship with God, our families, and our friends. It was a time of togetherness unlike any other. A time of reflection and a time of enjoyment. On Thanksgiving and Christmas, we reflected on how far we'd come and we enjoyed each other's company – and each other's food.

If your family is like mine, food is a big part of the celebration. Everyone wants to know what's on the menu and vies for inclusion of their favorite dish. When the day finally arrives and the table is set, the dinner spread is like a scene out of a movie (Soul Food to be exact) and food is e-v-e-r-y-w-h-e-r-e! I mean, the table is filled with turkey, ham, potato salad, green beans, yams, macaroni and cheese, greens, you name it and we have it. For dessert there are an assortment of cakes and pies – including grandma's famous sweet potato. To be honest, it's almost ridiculous how much food we have! There is so much food that you almost don't know where to start…or stop. Back in the day, I ate so much that I'd have to take a 1-2 hour break between dinner and dessert. There simply wasn't any room for anything else!

According to a 2000 study conducted by the National Institute of Child Health and Human Development (NICHD) and the National Institute of Diabetes and Digestive and Kidney Diseases (NIDDK), mine was not the only family that celebrated that way. In their studies it was determined that we are likely to gain an average of 1 pound in the 6 week period between Thanksgiving and New Year's Day. May not sound like a lot, but researchers also found that one year later, the participants in the study group did not lose any weight. In fact, they gained another 0.4 pounds making them 1.4 pounds heavier than the previous year. And, if you consider that this story is likely to repeat itself year after year, a 5'8' woman weighing 158 pounds today, could weigh 186 pounds 20 years from now. That extra 20 pounds that seemed to creep on, would move her from a normal weight to overweight. If she happened to pick up just an extra ½ pound a year, she'd weigh in at 197 pounds at the end of that 20 year period and for her height, 197 pounds is considered obese.

To make matters worse, although the *average* gain is only one pound, people who are already overweight tend to gain a lot more. A 2000 study by the USDA Human Nutrition Research Center on Aging found that overweight people gained five pounds or more during the holidays. I don't even have to do the math. You know this story would not end well.

## Tried and Tested

But this November, I was in a totally different mindset than the years before. I had lost 70 pounds and was down 100 pounds from my highest weight. At first, the thought of Thanksgiving dinner scared me. I had been controlling my portions and eating healthier foods, but I had never faced a test of my will like this. With all the distractions, would I really stick to my exercise plan? With so much high calorie, good tasting soul food in abundance, would I really be able to exercise restraint? I honestly didn't know the answers to these questions. I had done well all year, but this was a totally different ball game. I had to be honest with myself about where I was (mentally) and what I could reasonably commit to doing. If you want to be successful in this area, you will need to do the same.

Clearly, the "eat until you're stuffed" approach was not a good idea. But where was the balance? After all, the holidays only came once per year and this was the only time I had this spread of food on one day. These were some of my favorite foods and I wanted to enjoy them! At the same time, I didn't want to risk ruining all of my progress. I knew that one day did not cancel out everything. I knew that there were defining moments and slippery slopes. If I went too far, I could start something that I was ill-prepared to finish. If I pigged out, I could unbridle the lack of self-control I had just learned to constrain. If I gave myself too much freedom, I knew I would regret my decision later.

I decided that if I were to have any chance of making it through the holiday season without gaining weight, I had to have a plan.

> *"Success depends upon previous preparation and without such preparation there is sure to be failure."*
> *~Confucius*

I followed a similar approach as I did in the goal setting process earlier in the year. I started by asking myself some questions:

1. ***Are you going to work out? Or are you going to take some time "off"?*** If I skipped my workouts, I'd need to eat less than I normally did. I was already finding that I had to be more active to burn the same amount of calories as before because I now weighed less. The holidays would be challenging enough; I didn't want the added pressure of having to cut back. I decided that I would stick to my workout schedule to offset some of the tasty treats!

2. ***If you will work out, what type of exercise will you do?*** Fortunately this was an easy question for me to answer. I was already doing an at-home DVD and I resolved to continue it through the holidays. If you typically workout at the gym and you'll be away from home, remember that you will be out of your element and may not have access to a gym. If you have DVDs, take them with you. Other options: Look up workouts online or look for the fitness channel on cable TV. If all else fails, jumping jacks, pushups, jogging in place, jumping rope, lunges, and squats are easy to do anywhere.

3. ***When will you workout?*** At first I thought I would have plenty of time to get my workouts in, after all, I would be off from work. But then I realized that socializing and shopping with family and friends would take up most of the day. Once we let the good times roll, I wouldn't want to stop. I decided that the best approach was to get the workout in, and out of the way, before breakfast.

4. ***What is your goal?*** Understanding what typically happened during the holidays and knowing how hard I had worked all year, I decided that my goal would be to maintain my current weight. For a recovering "foodaholic", that would be an impressive victory! If you would like to continue along the path of weight loss, know this: It's not impossible to lose weight during the holidays. You just have to be willing to stick to your guns. If you

want a little freedom, that's ok, just resolve to maintain and get back to business within a few days.

5. ***What are your boundaries?*** Might seem like a foreign concept with it being the season of indulgence, but I knew that boundaries were necessary if I wanted to stay on track with my goals. A little freedom is okay, utter disregard for boundaries is not. Even though I had decided in advance to indulge, I wanted to do so within reason and so will you. Decide how many plates you'll get at dinner now (hint: the answer is 1) and choose what items are must haves (for me it was yams, mac and cheese, and cake) and forgo or get super small portions of the rest.

6. ***When will you get back to business?*** I had decided that it was okay to go off plan, but I needed a firm timeline for when I would get back to my normal routine. Otherwise, it would be slippery slope city. I recommend that your "vacation" not exceed 3 days. The longer you're "off" the harder it is to get back on track. Remember that even when you are off plan, you're not going hog wild.

---

### Quick Tips

- Create a workout schedule for the holidays. Decide on days, times, and workouts.
- Decide on "must have" foods and commit to eating reasonable portions. Stick to your one plate limit. Yes, you can have dessert within reason.
- Decide on a "stop date." This is the day that you will go back to eating on plan. It should be no more than 3 days since you went off plan unless you are willing to run the risk of gaining weight.

---

Taking the time to come up with a plan made me feel a whole lot better going into Thanksgiving. I would be able to have some freedom without getting completely off track. By thinking about what I was going to do ahead of time, I would avoid making rash decisions that were incongruent with my goals and end up paying the price later.

## Date with Destiny

When November 27th rolled around, it was much harder than I imagined. Temptations were all around to skip my workouts and eat more than I said I would. Of the two, eating reasonably was definitely the bigger challenge. The aroma of the food filled my nostrils and it all looked so good. My first instinct was to abandon my philosophy of restraint and eat everything in sight.

Family and friends didn't help the situation much either. I hadn't seen a few of them in quite a while and they were stunned by my transformation. I was flooded with compliments and questions about what I had been doing. Then I heard things like "girl, well you go ahead and enjoy yourself, you've earned it!" and "you're not dieting today are you?" I started to think that my attempt to exercise restraint was making some people uncomfortable. So, to ease their discomfort, they encouraged me to let go - after all *it is the holidays*. I could always get back to my healthy eating and exercise plan in the New Year along with everyone else.

I started to crumble under the pressure. I still exercised restraint, but I let go more than I should have. I was disappointed in myself because I didn't stick to my plan. I gained 3 pounds.

## Back to the Drawing Board

During the holidays and at other times through the year, our environment plays a big part in how we behave. No one is an island. We are all constantly influencing and being influenced. The most dominant, most consistent forces – whether they be good or evil – will almost always win. If you constantly surround yourself with drug addicts, chances are at some point, you will try drugs too. If the women in your circle are promiscuous, some of their attitudes about sex and relationships will probably rub off on you. If your father was a workaholic, chances are you will struggle with work/life balance. If you hang out with people that make unhealthy food choices on the norm, the risk that you will also make unhealthy food choices is high. Sometimes the progression is a conscious one and at other times, the subtle cues that we receive from the environment enter our subconscious mind over time and influence our resolve.

The ray of sunshine was that I was able to get back on track. Thanksgiving came and went and I was back to my old routine. I exercised extra hard in an attempt to make up for my overindulgence and focused on eating fruits and veggies. As I reflected on the situation, I realized that most of what I had gained wasn't fat. Yes, I had overindulged, but not 10,500 calories worth! In that moment I was thankful for all of the research I had done about calories. It gave me the assurance that all was not lost. I just had to get re-focused. Within a week, I was back to my pre-Thanksgiving weight.

> ### Quick Tip
> Whenever you see large fluctuations on the scale, do a sanity check. A pound of fat is equivalent to 3,500 calories. If you didn't eat 3,500 calories over and above your target, what you are seeing on the scale is only temporary. Consumption of a big meal, excess salt intake, water retention, constipation and hormonal changes can cause weight fluctuations. Don't freak out!

> *"At the end of each day, you should play back the tapes of your performance. The results should either applaud you or prod you."*
> ~ *Jim Rohn*

What is the big difference between successful people and unsuccessful people? Successful people, in any arena, take the time to self-reflect and self-evaluate. They don't always execute perfectly, but they are willing to stop and take stock of what went well and what could be done differently next time to get better results.

I didn't execute perfectly on my plan but I did much better than I would have done a year prior. Most importantly, I learned a valuable lesson: I had to make some changes in my circle.

No, it wasn't about de-friending anyone, disowning members of my family, or even skipping Thanksgiving dinner. It wasn't about changing them, it was about changing the level of *influence* they had on me. In this area of life, I couldn't take my cues from them. I would have to be the leader. The signals on what to do or what not to do would have to come from a different place. I would have to come off of auto-pilot and not just do what felt good or what everyone else was doing. I would have to dare to be different and be willing to deal with the attention and drama that may come along with it.

Whenever we change, we unconsciously disrupt the lives of those around us. The truth is this: Good changes, don't always feel good to our friends and family and that is what creates the rub. Let's face it: the fact that you're no longer the same person sometimes makes *you* uncomfortable! It only stands to reason that your friends will experience a degree of discomfort as well. For some, your decision to change may trigger feelings of guilt because they realize that they should be making changes too. In others, the change in dynamic may lead to feelings of insecurity because many of your shared activities revolved around food and they wonder where your relationship will now stand. And as you begin to make progress, some will try to impose their own beliefs on you or even sabotage your progress. Perhaps the ones you would least expect, like your husband, mom, or best friend. Still, the most dominant, most consistent forces – whether they are good or evil – will almost always win. The question then is - who will be the most dominant, most consistent force – *you or them?*

You have to be stronger. You have to be wiser. You must be willing to endure criticism. You must be willing to stand up and fight. Fight for the freedom to make your own choices. Fight for a healthier body. Fight for your new life.

Reflection Points

1. How has your environment influenced you?
2. How have you influenced others in your circle?

# Chapter 15 - 80/20

> *"Failure is simply the opportunity to begin again, this time more intelligently."*
> ~Henry Ford

I entered 2009 with excitement and optimism. I didn't accomplish all that I had set out to do over the holidays, but I walked away from the experience with something even more valuable. In my time of anxiety, the 80/20 rule was born.

<u>Ah Ha Moment</u>

Up until the holiday season, I had allowed myself one treat day per week, usually Saturday. Even on my treat day, I didn't just eat whatever I wanted. My treat normally amounted to a nice dinner – a lean steak and baked potato with a small pat of butter or a half of a chocolate lava cake. This tremendous focus allowed me to reach my goal quickly, but it had very little "grace" built in. The holidays taught me that there was a way to strike a balance. In the entire six week period, I gained 5 pounds and just a few days into the New Year, I had lost it all. Again, very little of it was fat, so once I got back to my normal routine, the puffiness and bloating disappeared.

Now that is not to say that I was okay with gaining 5 pounds over the holidays. It was not my ideal outcome and I intended to do better going forward. But, the beautiful thing was that it wasn't the end of the world either. I allowed myself more freedom than I did in the previous 9 months and my new size 10/12 frame survived. That got me to thinking. Maybe I didn't have to limit myself to one treat day. Maybe I could introduce a little more freedom in my diet if I worked them into my plan.

I had been managing the same calorie target every day which worked well except for on the weekends. The weekends were when I was typically out and about with my friends and food was always on the agenda. By this time I was fairly skilled at identifying foods that aligned with my meal plan, but it was getting tough, really tough to always choose the "right" thing. Clearly I didn't want to go back to all of my old habits but I did want to live a little. I started playing with the numbers and I was surprised by what I saw.

Fuzzy Math

At my current weight and activity level, my daily calorie target was 1,800. Since there were 7 days in a week that meant I had a total of 12,600 calories in my "bank" per week. If I allocated 50% of those calories Monday through Thursday and 50% to Friday through Sunday, I could have my cake and eat it too, literally!

*Here's how it worked out:*

**Average Calories per Day * Days per Week = Total Weekly Calorie Bank**

$$1800 * 7 = 12{,}600$$

**(Total Calorie Bank * 50%) ÷ 4 = Monday through Thursday Target**

$$(12{,}600 * 50\% = 6{,}300 \text{ total calories}) \div 4$$

$$= 1{,}575 \text{ calories per day}$$

**Remaining Calories ÷ 3 days = Weekend Daily Calorie Target**

$$(12,600 - 6,300) \div 3$$

$$= 2,100 \text{ calories per day}$$

My 80/20 plan for the typical week looked like this:

| Day | Target |
|-----------|--------|
| Monday | 1575 |
| Tuesday | 1575 |
| Wednesday | 1575 |
| Thursday | 1575 |
| Friday | 2100 |
| Saturday | 2100 |
| Sunday | 2100 |
| Total | 12600 |

I was so excited I could almost burst! There *was* a way to keep the weight off and enjoy some of my favorite foods. And the system was totally flexible; if there was a potluck at work on Wednesday or a friend's birthday dinner on Thursday, it still worked. All I had to do to stay on track was swap one of my weekend days with the day of the potluck or dinner.

Wednesday potluck:

| Day | Target |
|-----------|--------|
| Monday | 1575 |
| Tuesday | 1575 |
| Wednesday | 2100 |
| Thursday | 1575 |
| Friday | 1575 |
| Saturday | 2100 |
| Sunday | 2100 |
| Total | 12600 |

Thursday dinner:

| Day | Target |
|-----------|--------|
| Monday | 1575 |
| Tuesday | 1575 |
| Wednesday | 1575 |
| Thursday | 2100 |
| Friday | 2100 |
| Saturday | 2100 |
| Sunday | 1575 |
| Total | 12600 |

It was like discovering gold! I now had a clear plan that would allow me to have a mental and emotional break from trying to eat a near-perfect diet without ending up back at square one! I'll be straight with you --a part of me doubted if this would really work. I had been so hard and fast on that one treat day per week. I was scared that this new plan would backfire on me (even though it worked on paper). I mean, I was a recovering food addict; would this cause more harm than good?

Consistent Imperfection

The question I raised was a fair one. I could be opening Pandora's Box here. This 80/20 plan could set off a chain of events that would easily spiral out of control. I was scared. I didn't want to go back to the person I was. But still, I reasoned, I had to try it. After all, we were talking about the rest of my life here. Eating near-perfectly 6 days a week for the next 40 years was completely doable but not a whole lot of fun. I had to create a system that would work for me -- mentally, emotionally, and physically -- long-term and I believed this was it. It was a calculated risk; as long as I stuck to the plan, I would continue to beat this thing.

I was a nervous wreck my first few days under the 80/20 plan. I had to talk myself out of jumping on the scale nearly every day. I wanted so badly to know if it was working! Determined to see it through, I fought temptation like a bulldog and hid the scale at the bottom of my dirty clothes hamper – out of sight, out of mind. Finally, at the end of the week, I pulled out the scale. Once again, I took a deep breath and stepped on the scale. I closed my eyes. I was afraid to look down.

After what seemed like several minutes, I tilted my head downwards and opened my eyes. 164! I still weighed 164!! What a sigh of relief! It worked, it really worked!

Being consistently imperfect -- that is what it is all about. Don't believe the hype. You don't have to dot every "I" and cross every "T" every day. You *can* enjoy the foods you love without sabotaging your progress. I am a witness, if you work the 80/20 as designed, it works!

Reflection Points

1. What would your 80/20 plan look like?
2. How would it feel to be able to enjoy the foods you love (within reason) and still lose weight?

# PART III: LOOKING GOOD

"When you look good, you feel good."
~Maria Sharapova

# Chapter 16 - I Like the Mirror

"Karen!" I said as she walked by. "Yes?" she replied, sounding and looking confused. "Karen" then looked me dead in the eye as if she was trying to figure out who I was. Still looking puzzled she said "I know that voice but, but…" She was struggling to make sense of it all. I decided to bail her out. "Karen, it's me. It's Tamara." The look on her face was priceless. Shock, awe, excitement all at once. "Oh my gosh! I didn't even recognize you!" I smiled and said "I look a little different huh?" Her face said it all. I looked *a lot* different. It was a night and day difference.

Perfect Strangers

"Karen's" reaction was a pretty common one. I bore a resemblance to my former self, yet I looked so starkly different that it was difficult for people to process. The image people had grown to associate with me was no longer a valid one. Even though "Karen" and I had known each other for years, she walked right past me. Equally as entertaining was my family members' reactions; people that knew me for the 26 years before I gained the weight, walked by me without knowing who I was too. I guess after a while, people forget the old you. What you looked like prior to gaining weight just disappears from their memory banks. They may have forgotten, but the image of my slimmer, more confident self, had not vanished from my memory. I remembered her and I was glad to have her back!

> *"I love looking in the mirror and feeling good about what I see."*
> *~Heather Morris*

For the first time in 8 years, I was happy with how I looked. I liked my reflection in the mirror. I no longer cringed. I no longer had to suck things in. My clothes fit perfectly. Clothes in a size that I wasn't sure I would ever be able to wear again. I was back in the Misses section with "regular" folks; imagine that! I was amazed by how different the clothes looked and fit. Not just on the mannequin, but on me. I had style.

It wasn't just wearing a smaller size that made a difference. My chubby face was now slim. My arms and legs were smaller; my stomach flatter. I looked younger, much younger. Some people mistakenly thought I was still in my twenties. It felt good, so good! All the hard work had finally paid off. I was attractive to myself again.

I didn't realize how much of a toll being obese had taken on me. I had become strangely accustomed to my undesirable condition. It's like that bad smell that sometimes surfaces in the kitchen; maybe something in the fridge. At first you think, "Man, what is that? I've got to find it and throw it out!" But if you put it off long enough without taking action, your nose adjusts to the smell. The bad scent is still there, but it isn't noticeable to you anymore. Once acutely aware of how bad it smelled, you have now forgotten that it's even there! Occasionally something happens that reminds you. A friend or family member says you've put on weight. Your favorite outfit catches your eye and you remember how long it's been since you could last wear it. You take a long, hard look at yourself in the mirror. You hate your situation. It stinks. But you have become used to it...and you stay there. You stay in a place that you would rather not be. You remain bound.

But here's the thing: If you go outside, breathe in the fresh air, and come back in, your perspective changes. Once you spend enough time away from the stench and re-enter the house, you smell it again, that horrible, rotten smell. You resolve that you never, ever want to smell that scent again and take immediate action to ensure that your desire becomes a reality. But had you never ventured outside and experienced what life was like without the stench, you never would have realized what you were missing. That's how I was for 8 years, but no more. Now that I had ventured outside, I never ever wanted to be that person again. Not because I hated her, but because I was finally happy with me.

> *Happiness (noun):*
> *A mental or emotional state of well-being characterized by positive or pleasant emotions ranging from contentment to intense joy.*

New Life

But why was I happy? Was it just the fact that I was at my lowest weight in 8 years? Did I simply like what I saw in the mirror? Or was it that I looked so astonishingly different that my own family didn't recognize me? I certainly got a kick out of all of this, but no, I can't say that any of these things was ultimately responsible for my happiness. What was it then? What or who made me happy?

By this point, I had been blessed with a nice home in an up-and-coming neighborhood, drove a nice car, and was earning a nice income. I hadn't found Mr. Right, but I was okay with that. I figured he was on the way and would reveal himself at the proper time. So was it the fact that I was finally on track with my childhood dreams that made me happy? No. The truth is that I had all these things in 2006 - the same year I lost 40 pounds and regained 10 - and I wasn't happy then either.

Although we often hang our hopes for a better life on money, possessions, health, and beauty, scientific research has shown that these are only minor factors in the quest for happiness. For example, a study by Ed Diener from the University of Illinois[26] found that the wealthiest Americans – those earning more than $10 million annually – reported levels of personal happiness only slightly greater than the people who work for them (at significantly lower salaries I would presume). But you didn't need me to tell you that to know that it's true. Every day we hear stories of unhappy celebrities, CEOs, athletes, and artists. They have everything that money can buy but are still empty inside. To compensate, they cheat on their spouses or significant others, do drugs, work around the clock to accumulate more money, and participate in other self-destructive behaviors because they mistakenly believe that doing so will cure what ails them. What were they missing? What had *I* been missing?

For me, love was the missing piece of the puzzle. For years my heart was like a car on "E." I waited and waited on the side of the road for my true love, my rescuer to appear, but he never came. Don't get me wrong, there were many who stopped by, but they didn't have true love on their mind. Each time was a journey to nowhere and I constantly found myself back on the side of the road again, hurt and confused. When love didn't work, I threw myself into my career, thinking it could fill the void. It didn't. I ended up working a lot of long nights and still felt empty and unfulfilled. I yearned for that special love, but I could never seem to find it.

I am reminded of a situation in the Bible that talks about true love. A notorious group wanted to trick The Teacher by asking a controversial question: Which is the most important commandment? The Teacher replied that the first and greatest commandment is to love God with "all your heart, all your soul, and all of your mind." But then there was another, in The Teacher's own words, "equally important" commandment: "Love your neighbor as yourself." He concluded His thought-provoking answer by saying that all of the commandments hinged on these two. Interesting.

I spent a lot of time in church services as a child, teenager and young adult. I knew that loving God completely was of paramount importance. I understood that no matter how badly they irked my nerves, I needed to find the strength to love my neighbor. What had escaped me was that I was to love my neighbors (family, friends, co-workers, acquaintances, and enemies) *as I loved myself.* That implied that self-love was a prerequisite to properly loving others. In all the years that I heard and read that passage, that part of the message never sank in.

I also found it interesting that, to The Teacher, self-love was a given. It was not something that some had and others didn't. No, a love of self was something we were all born with - original manufacturer equipment. If you think about it, we all have a powerful instinct of self-preservation and self-fulfillment. We want to live a long, happy life and we want someone "nice" to share our lives with. We want "nice" clothes to wear, "nice" shoes and a "nice-sized" closet to put them in. We dream of living in a "nice" home in a "nice" neighborhood, paid for with a "nice" income from a "nice" job that we work or business we own where we are surrounded with "nice" co-workers. We all want to live with a sense of purpose. We all want some form of the "good life "with "good" friends, food, and frequent vacations. All of these desires are a form of self-love, a deep longing to move away from pain and propel ourselves towards happiness. But here is where I and those celebrities I talked about missed it: it takes more than money, possessions, accomplishments, and things to feel fulfilled. Much more.

Fulfillment comes when we are living on purpose and in a way that is consistent with what we value most. The extra weight that we carry around – whether it be physical, emotional, or psychological – limits our ability to do that. Whenever we are not being our authentic self, we won't feel complete because the extra weight distorts our view. We no longer see ourselves the way God sees us. Instead our view becomes a contorted one, like one you would see in one of those trick mirrors at the state fair. If we don't know how to love ourselves and address what isn't working in our lives, we will feel like a failure no matter how much it looks like we've accomplished. In an attempt to make those feelings go away, we medicate our pain with something. My medication of choice was food.

For years, I had been unconsciously medicating my pain - the failed relationships, the hole in my heart, and the feelings of inadequacy- with food. I wallowed in self-pity. I played the victim. It was always someone else's fault. I was powerless. But now my viewpoint was changing. I no longer saw myself as a victim, but as a victor.

I was happy because I was finally learning the proper context of love: love God, love myself, and love others. It was a package deal, not an either or proposition. I also came to understand that achievements and things weren't enough to keep me in a state of happiness, neither were my relationships with other people. Whenever I relied on someone other than God and myself to make me feel loved, I was setting myself up for disappointment.

To be able to be loved, I had to love and respect myself as much as I did others. Finally, I was in a position to do that. I'm still a work in progress, but I can honestly say that for the first time in my life, I am on the road to true happiness. Are you?

Reflection Points

1.  Are you happy? Why or why not?
2.  How would your life change if you finally and forever lost the weight?

26.  Psychologytoday.com, 2008

# Chapter 17 - Something New – Pride

hopeless adj.

1. Having no hope; despairing.

2. Offering no hope; bleak.

3. Incurable.

4. Having no possibility of solution; **impossible**.

<u>Hope Deferred</u>

As a child, I was a big believer in possibilities. When my mom and dad separated, I held on to hope for years that they would find their way back to each other again --despite an abundance of evidence to the contrary. And, even though the idea of carrying on conversations with complete strangers and speaking up in public terrified me, I believed I would one day occupy the positions of President and CEO. I didn't have a lot of good examples of successful marriages, but I still believed in love and remained optimistic that when I married, mine would last. But then, the idea of impossibilities began to invade my space. My parents never did get back together. I was having trouble breaking through the glass ceiling at work. And, after being in and seeing others go through a string of bad relationships, I was beginning to lose faith in love and marriage. Worst of all, I had lost faith in me.

> *"What happens to a dream deferred?*
>
> *Does it dry up*
>
> *like a raisin in the sun?*
>
> *Or fester like a sore--*
>
> *And then run?*
>
> *Does it stink like rotten meat?*
>
> *Or crust and sugar over--*
>
> *like a syrupy sweet?*
>
> *Maybe it just sags*
>
> *like a heavy load.*
>
> *Or does it explode?"*
>
> *~Langston Hughes*

The Book of Wisdom says that "hope deferred makes the heart sick" and I was in the infirmary. When my life went in directions I didn't expect, I stopped expecting good things to happen to me. I began anticipating roadblocks and failures. The more I wanted something, the more it seemed to evade me. The longer I waited, the worse the situation looked. The more I longed to be fulfilled, the emptier I felt. Worst of all, I felt powerless to change any of it. With every setback, real or imagined, I lost a little more faith in my ability to change, to grow, to become. Eventually the feelings of hopelessness came to a head and I was overwhelmed by it all. I started to believe my situation was incurable, that I was a lost cause.

Trying and failing to lose weight over and over again only exacerbated those feelings. Just when I started to believe I was turning the corner, I would fall off the bandwagon. I would give in to a craving or decide to skip a workout, not realizing that each time I failed to follow through on a promise I made to myself I was eroding my self-confidence. Instead of building myself up, I was constantly tearing myself down. I was stuck in my own personal hell with no way out. I was living life without hope…until now.

> *"We are products of our past, but we don't have to be prisoners of it."*
> ~ *Rick Warren*

The New Me

But when October of 2008 rolled around, I had changed from the inside out. Being able to weather the ups and downs of the first 10 months of my new lifestyle renewed my confidence in my ability to change.

As I looked back over the year, I was proud of myself for all of the adjustments I made.

- When I realized evening workouts weren't working, I started going to bed earlier so I could exercise before work.
- When I discovered that my eating habits were self-destructive, I taught myself how to eat healthily and in reasonable portions.
- I accepted the fact that I wasn't perfect and allowed myself some freedom in my diet within proper boundaries.
- Sodas and sweets surprisingly moved from regular treats to occasional indulgences.
- I taught myself how to conquer my cravings; I became a mindful eater.
- I went from never working out to working out 6 days a week and I actually enjoyed it!

The journey I had embarked upon encouraged me to believe in possibilities again. It *was* possible; I *could* change. You can too.

> *"No matter who you are, no matter what you did, no matter where you've*
> *come from, you can always change; become a better version of yourself."*
> ~Madonna

## 3 TIPS TO COMBAT HOPELESSNESS

1. ***Let go of unrealistic expectations.*** While it was good to be young and ambitious, I had no concept of what the real world was like. I assumed college would be just like high school (relatively easy). I thought that there would be an abundance of job offers when I graduated and that education alone was enough to command a comfortable salary. I even believed I could retire at 40! Now I'm not saying it's impossible to reach these goals, but 1) I hadn't done my research to understand what types of sacrifices I would have to make to achieve the results I wanted and 2) I put way too much pressure on myself! When things didn't pan out like I planned, my self-esteem took a huge blow and I struggled to snap out of it.

   The concept of realistic expectations also applies to your weight loss goals. It takes a different level of commitment to lose 10 pounds in one month than it does to lose it in two or three. Do the work to understand what it takes physically, mentally, and emotionally to achieve what you desire, then do a sanity check – "Am I willing to make that sacrifice?"

   Oh and once you start, be careful not to expect too much too soon. Starting a new workout regimen one week and expecting to see a total transformation the following, isn't realistic. Change takes time.

2. ***Stop being your worst critic.*** One of my mistakes was allowing my shortcomings to overshadow my strengths. We all have strengths *and* weaknesses. Break out a piece of paper and force yourself to list an equal number of strengths and weaknesses. Be honest in your assessment of your shortcomings, but also think about the things you've been complimented on, what you've been

told sets you apart from others, and previous personal victories. If you have trouble coming up with strengths, which is very common, get help from your most supportive friends, family members and co-workers. Ask them to tell you what they think you are good at. You will be surprised by how quickly your list builds and your confidence level grows. Post your brag sheet (strengths) and start developing a plan to address your areas of opportunity with realistic and attainable short-term goals. Then take it one day at a time, celebrating your victories and learning from your mistakes.

3. ***Focus on progress, not perfection.*** God doesn't expect us to be perfect, so why do we? Be patient with yourself. You may not achieve every life goal within the timeframe that you planned. You may not ever have the perfect body or the perfect relationship. But here's the thing: a perfect life only exists in movies. It's an allusive goal that many of us strive to attain at the risk of our peace and our sanity. Let it go.

I challenge you to focus on progress, not perfection, in life and in your quest to be healthy and fit. Caving in to peer pressure at one meal doesn't spell impending doom and disaster. Struggling through the first workout doesn't mean that the regimen is too hard and can't be done. You must come to the realization that everyone – including you – is human. As long as we are in these earthly bodies, we will make mistakes, but mistakes (or the absence of them) do not define who we are. Contrary to how it may feel, your performance *does not* determine your worth. Missing the mark does not make you a failure; it simply means you – like everyone else – are a work in progress. Relax!

> *"People throw away what they could have by insisting on perfection, which they cannot have, and looking for it where they will never find it."*
> *~Edith Schaeffer*

<u>Reflection Points</u>
1. What unrealistic expectations have been holding you captive?
2. How often do you identify and celebrate your victories?
3. Are you a perfectionist? If so, how is that mindset making it more difficult to reach your goals?

# Chapter 18 – Inhaling Power

> *"Perplexity is the beginning of knowledge."*
> *~ Kahlil Gibran*
>
> *"Knowledge is power."*
> *~Francis Bacon*

Duped. Hoodwinked. Bamboozled. These were the feelings that were typically associated with my weight loss efforts. Things generally started off promisingly, with me dropping 5+ pounds in the first week, but shortly thereafter my progress seemed to stall. 1 pound, 2 pounds on a good week, was more the norm and that just wasn't good enough. With all of the hard work I was putting into all of this – skipping meals, feeling like someone was gnawing a hole in my stomach, sweating like crazy and looking like a fool in the gym – why was I getting such poor results? Maybe I cheated a little bit here and there but surely that wasn't enough to ruin everything! Or was it?

Most of the time, it just didn't seem worth it. Why was this so hard? Other people lost weight so effortlessly. What was I doing wrong? All of these were questions I found myself asking over and over again without ever reaching a sensible conclusion…until now. They say that knowledge is power and finally I was a force to be reckoned with. I was in control of my destiny. I was unstoppable.

## Total Responsibility

I've often said that weight loss is simple, but not easy. To this day I stick by that assertion. It's simple in that the formula is straightforward – eat less and move more. But how much less is enough? How much more counts? Those were the pieces of the puzzle that I was missing. Then I learned the importance of tidbits like calculating my basil metabolic rate, estimating the number of calories I burned in a typical workout, choosing appropriate portion sizes and spotting common diet derailers. Without these insights, there remained a sizeable gap between what I *thought* I was doing and what I was *actually* accomplishing. How frustrating!

Now that I really understood what it took to be successful at weight loss, my frustrations were gone. I knew what was required to get the results that I wanted and approximately how long it would take – no more guesswork. When I veered off course, I understood that it wasn't the end of the world; I knew how to get back on track. If the outcome felt short of my expectations, I knew precisely what behavior gaps to look for, because it wasn't the fault of the workout or the meal plan. I was the one to blame. This time, I was taking 100% responsibility for the results – good, bad or indifferent.

Taking full responsibility did not mean that I acted as though there were not outside factors influencing the outcomes in my life. It simply meant that I refused to give those factors the final say. I was the captain of the ship, not my boss and his unrealistic demands, my fickle feelings or even the numbers on my digital scale. I couldn't always choose my circumstances, but I could always choose how I responded to them.

I would no longer allow myself to be bossed around by what others said or did or even those irrational things I said to myself. I strived to be grounded in truth and let truth be my measuring stick. I challenged myself to look at the facts and nothing but the facts, because unlike me, my feelings, and well-intentioned friends, family members, and acquaintances, the facts didn't lie. I was either cutting it or I wasn't. If I wasn't cutting it, I needed to go back to the drawing board and figure out where I went wrong. No more blaming. No more complaining. The responsibility of finding a way to succeed was mine and mine alone.

Because I stopped making excuses, I moved from being problem to solution oriented. That solution orientation made me hungry for knowledge, not just in terms of the science of weight loss but the psychological aspects as well. I came to realize that developing the proper mindset and learning how to control my emotions was equally, if not more important, than understanding how to calculate my daily calorie deficit. Changing my way of thinking changed everything. It can do the same for you.

## 5 FACTS YOU MAY NOT KNOW ABOUT WEIGHT LOSS

1. **Motivation Fades.** Listen to me. There is nothing wrong with you. You are not a special case. We *all* have moments of indifference, discouragement, or frustration. Therefore, it is important to create an environment that will be there to keep you going or pick you up when you are down. If you are a person that finds inspiration in quotes or pictures, then put these around the house to help you maintain motivation. Place them on your fridge, on your desk, on your night table, wherever you think might help you. Some people find that vision boards (a board on which you display images that represent whatever you want to be, do or have in your life), going public with their goals and plans on Facebook, joining a team weight loss challenge, or creating and posting a "contract for success" with themselves helps keep them on the straight and narrow. The method you use is not important. What is important is that you find what works for you and use it consistently. One of my favorite quotes on this subject: "People often say that motivation doesn't last. Well, neither does bathing that's why we recommend it daily." – Zig Ziglar

2. **Your willpower isn't fixed. Like muscle, discipline can be built.** Saying that weight loss is "too hard" or "I just don't have

any willpower" is a cop out. It is our subtle way of saying that we are powerless to change and that just isn't true. In reality, we have the ability to change any time we choose but it's going to take work. Just as the little girl that dreams of becoming a world-class athlete must practice building her endurance, speed and strength, we must practice exercising discipline daily. The more we do it, the stronger we become.

Sure, some may be naturally more disciplined than others but isn't that true in every facet of life? Some are gifted at math and others English. Some are creative souls and others logical thinkers. Some are spontaneous and others planners. We can't afford to look at the disciplined people in our lives with envy. Instead, we need to study what they do and figure out how we can replicate it. Ask yourself, what can I learn from "Jessica" that will make my life better?

We all have strength zones and areas that challenge us. When something isn't strength for us, it doesn't mean that we can just throw up our hands and give up. Just like everything else that we weren't good at the first time around, we have to roll up our sleeves and get to work. We have to be persistent. We must accept that we will make mistakes. Here is the beauty of it all: we all start out as beginners, but if we keep it, we eventually become competent, then proficient. Who knows, if we're fortunate, we may even become an expert. Practice doesn't make perfect, but it does produce progress.

Always remember this process takes time; it doesn't happen overnight. Just as it takes time to learn a new language, excel in a new position at work, or adjust to a new relationship, succeeding at weight loss takes time.

3. ***Superficial goals always yield temporary results.*** Although fitting into a smaller size is appealing, for most of us it's not enough to spark a permanent change. It may motivate us for a few days, weeks, or even months, but rarely is it enough to keep us committed for life. This is why it is so common to lose weight

and regain it. In order to succeed long term, you need will power *and* why power and your why must be tied to what you value most.

Author John Maxwell says it like this: "Once your commitment is based on your values, you have no problem sustaining it. Values are what drive your choices; they transcend your talents and skills and they stand up under the tests of adversity. Commitment based on something other than solid values usually is a house of cards; when the wind kicks up, the house comes down." Having lost weight and regained it twice, I am a witness to John's comments. I stuck to the plan for a while, but eventually grew tired of it. The idea of enjoying my favorite foods and avoiding the embarrassment of the gym soon outweighed my desire to be thinner. Without tying my goals to my values, my weight loss strategy was a house of cards just waiting for a good wind to knock it down. (By the way: the wind always comes, the question is will we be ready for it?)

By values I am referring to the people, places, ideals, abilities and things that are <u>most important </u>to you, not the things that are sort of kind of important. I'm talking about what you don't want to live without, what gets you out of bed in the morning, what makes you tick.

Is it:

- Your spouse?
- Your children?
- Your faith?
- Achieving goals you have set for yourself?
- Being active in the community?
- Being a person of excellence?
- Being a good steward?
- Traveling?
- Making a meaningful contribution at work?

- The idea of enjoying a relaxing and drama free retirement?
- Freedom to live, move, do as you please?

Chances are there are several things on this list that you value. It's important though, that you identify what you value most – your top 5. Think of it like this, if you had to live the rest of your life on the basis of 5 values -and only 5- what would you chose as your life's guiding principles? What couldn't you risk living without?

Now ask yourself:

- Am I living in a way that is consistent with these values?
- Is my current health status and level of fitness helping me or hurting me?
- What am I prepared to do about it?

4. **It's not enough to know, you have to be motivated enough to do.** Motivation is defined as "the reason or reasons one has for acting or behaving in a particular way." When a person is truly motivated, they don't just have a desire for something, they are willing to act and they follow through. After years of being unmotivated, my doctor helped me uncover my motivation by invoking what psychologists call the pain vs. pleasure principle.

What is the pain vs. pleasure principle? Well, some people are more naturally motivated towards pleasure (the thought of spending time with their children, enjoying retirement, traveling the world) while others are more motivated away from pain (having to start taking insulin or blood pressure medication, going up another dress or pant size, or not being able to play with their kids due to a lack of energy). The trick is to find out which one- "Towards Pleasure" or "Away From Pain"- is more compelling to you in terms of your values and to focus on that.

*If you are pleasure-oriented, ask yourself how your life will be better. "What positive impact will losing the weight have on my values?"*

Create a compelling picture for yourself that is rich in detail of how your life will be better.

- Would you be able to play with your kids without getting winded? What would that feel like?
- Would you have more energy to serve in the community? With that energy, what would you be able to accomplish?
- Would you be more alert and productive at work? How would that position you for success?
- Would you feel better about yourself? How would that translate into how you interact with others?
- Because you are healthier and physically fit, would you have a better quality of life in retirement? Where would you be able to go and what would you be able to do?

*If you are more motivated by moving away from pain ask yourself: "So if I don't lose the weight, or if I continue to get heavier and heavier, what will stay the same or what could I potentially lose that I value?"*

- Will you not be able to play with your kids very long after school because you lack the energy? How will it feel if you have to endure that for another year?
- Will you feel drained and lethargic after a full day's work like you do today? Can you see yourself continuing to live that way?
- Will your self-image suffer? Will you be displeased when you look in the mirror even though you know in your heart that you are more than your size?
- Based on your family history and habits, will you likely end up on blood pressure medication, have to go on dialysis, or end up taking insulin? What type of experience will that be?

- Could you find yourself unable to fulfill your life purpose because you lack the stamina to do so? How would it feel to leave this earth with that call unfulfilled?
- Could you find yourself living in an assisted living facility in retirement instead of traveling the world like you planned? How would it feel to work 40-50 years and then spend your retirement this way?

I think you get the idea. The question is which one compels you to action – the thought of gaining something or losing something? For me – it was the prospect of losing something – my quality of life. I strongly value my independence and being confronted with the possibility of battling sickness and disease for the rest of my life completely changed my perspective. Having seen the havoc that heart disease, blood pressure issues, and kidney disease had on my family was just the motivation I needed. I wanted the cycle of sickness and disease to end. I couldn't let the same thing happen to me.

Here is the thing: everyone is different. The question is what will motivate you? How will your life be better if you lose the weight or worse if you don't? It's not something we like to think about, but it's crucial that we stop living on autopilot and seriously consider the consequences of our actions or inactions. Cultivate this picture until it gives you a clear sense of purpose. Once you have a clear picture, you are much more likely to take and sustain the necessary action.

---

**Please Note:**

*This exercise is not about creating fear. There are clearly consequences – good and bad – to our actions or inactions. Every day we plant seeds that will produce a harvest in the immediate or not so immediate future. This exercise is simply about looking ahead and seeing how those seeds either help create the life we want or push us further away. It's simply a matter of forecasting the positive or negative consequences of our actions or inactions and determining which approach is mostly likely to motivate us.*

---

Having a clear picture is important because there often is no immediate consequence if we choose not to change. You aren't confronted with the consequences of not working to develop your interpersonal and leadership skills until you miss out on the promotion. You don't understand the importance of openness and communication until your spouse files for divorce. You don't realize how important finding time to network is until you lose your job and find yourself short on contacts. Impulsive spending isn't really a problem until you reach the point of having more month than money and are struggling to pay your bills and save for retirement. Perhaps if we instantly suffered a heart attack or went into a diabetic coma after missing a workout or binging over the weekend, we would learn from the experience and wouldn't dare repeat it. But because we don't suffer immediate consequences, we are lulled into a state of inaction – until we get a wakeup call or it's too late.

We make our choices and our choices ultimately make us. We can choose to keep saying that we don't have time to manage our health, but we can't choose the consequences of that decision. If we choose not to act, of one thing we can be sure: chances are we aren't going to like it.

5. ***Weight management is a daily, lifelong process.*** This may have been one of the most eye-opening revelations I have had during the course of my journey. Weight management isn't a "set it and forget it" type of thing. Just like every other area of our lives - careers, relationships, social networks, and household finances – our weight has to be *constantly* managed. Your calorie target at 200 pounds isn't the same as it is at 180 pounds; for every 15-20 pounds you lose, you need to go back and recalculate. Similarly, the fitter you become the fewer calories you burn during exercise; you must continue to challenge yourself with new routines of increasing complexity to get results. To make matters even more interesting, the world of fitness is constantly evolving and inspiring new (or old) trends. Concepts like high-intensity interval training made popular by the likes of

*Insanity*, *P90X* and *CrossFit*, are a recent phenomenon, replacing traditional (and in my opinion boring) cardio. Bodyweight training and group training (vs. one-on-one personal training) are also making a comeback possibly inspired by a very tight economy. My point is the only thing that is constant is change. This is another reason why traditional dieting doesn't work: you have to have a plan that is strong enough to stand the test of time (you may have another 20-50 years to live you know) and flexible enough to adapt to your ever changing lifestyle. You must be curious; constantly learning and adapting, trying new things. Your health and fitness plan should evolve and grow over time in the same way that your life changes and evolves. If it doesn't, you start to lose ground and eventually you are right back where you started. Don't let that be your story.

Perplexity is the beginning of knowledge. Explore solutions and open your mind to the truth. In the end, truth will set you free.

Reflection Points

1. What are your top 5 values? Are you living in alignment with those values?
2. Are you motivated by going away from pain or towards pleasure? How can you use that to your advantage?

## Chapter 19 - Love This Thing Called "Confidence"

I knew I would never hear from him again but I waited anyway. Probably a good 10-15 minutes. Up until that point the conversations with "Michael" had been great; he even told me I was sexy and beautiful. His romantic charm, engaging personality and level of attentiveness actually made me feel that way. I loved the way I felt when I talked to him – like a school girl with a serious crush. It was a feeling I hadn't had in a long time. I wanted to hold on to it, but I could see it slipping away.

<u>Playing Defense</u>

I had encountered so many losers online that I was beginning to think that special person would never find me. I ran into scam artists, married men that posed as if they were single, and guys that were on the rebound from bad relationships. Occasionally I met what seemed to be a good guy, but after a couple of dates we knew that we weren't what each other was looking for, and parted ways. "Michael" and I had hit it off so well on the phone; I wanted to believe that this time would be different. What I thought was a dream come true was really a nightmare.

"Michael" eventually caught on to the fact that my online dating profile only had headshot pictures. He started bugging me for a full body picture – so that he could "see just how sexy I was." Every time he asked, I tried to switch subjects. For a while there, I got away with it, but he was persistent. Finally, he put his foot down - "I know you have a picture of yourself in your phone! Hang up and send it to me, then I'll call you right back." I knew I was cornered. According to his pictures, he was the tall, dark, handsome, athletic type and I knew what was going to happen next. I hung up, sent the picture, and never heard from "Michael" again.

A similar scenario played out a few more times during my 8 years of being overweight. Each time it stung like someone was pouring peroxide into my open wound. It was a painful reminder – I was no longer attractive to the type of guy that was attractive to me.

In my teenage and young adult years, I had been tall and slim. Sure, there were guys that preferred a woman with "a little more meat on her bones," but I still attracted my fair share of men. Now feeling like I didn't measure up was a regular occurrence. I hated that feeling.

I decided that I never wanted to feel that way again. I added head-to-toe pictures to my profile thinking that guys would opt-out and save us both the trouble. I adjusted my expectations – if he was my type and showed genuine interest, he had to be just playing games. After all, what did he see in me that the others didn't? I erected a wall – I wouldn't open myself up to that disappointment again. Soon I exited the dating scene all together. I had to protect my heart --and my dignity.

It's a Man's World

A dear friend of mine once said to me emphatically, "Men determine the standard of beauty." What a powerful statement. May sound crazy, but think about it. At a young age, a lot of emphasis is placed on how a little girl looks, dresses, and how she carries herself, all with the intention of teaching her how to be "ladylike." If the little girl looks or acts in a way that is inconsistent with the ideal, she is labeled a "tom boy" and is promptly coached to conform. As she grows older, the focus intensifies; it's not just about being ladylike anymore but attracting a "good man." Attracting that man, we are taught, largely comes down to appearance. The media caters to men and reinforces their definition of beauty – a pretty face and thin figure. Without even realizing it, we start to internalize these messages and begin to confuse our perceived level of beauty with our worth and value, not just in the dating arena but in every area of life.

I applied for promotions at work and was turned down time and time again. I was intellectually capable. I met all the stated job requirements. I had gone over-and-beyond and volunteered for stretch assignments. I had taken my team from a struggling to a performing one. What was I missing? What else should I have done? Where did I miss the mark? Despite asking repeatedly, the male leadership team never provided a legitimate answer to that question. And when you don't get answers, you jump to conclusions – conclusions that may or may not be valid.

I started to doubt my abilities. Maybe I wasn't ready? Maybe I needed to go somewhere else and start over? Maybe I wasn't good enough? I was feeling stuck; suffocated. I started to shut down. When questions were asked in meetings, I kept my opinions to myself. When I normally would have gone above and beyond, I was content with being average. I mean, what was the point? I didn't measure up, *again*.

But once I shed the weight - mentally, emotionally and physically - my perspective changed. I didn't wait for opportunity to knock. I busted down the door.

> *"Luck is what happens when preparation meets opportunity."*
> — *Lucius Annaeus Seneca*

## Divine Intervention

In January of 2009, just three months after reaching a healthy weight, I was asked to go to Charlotte, NC to assist with interviews for our newest location. A year prior I may have been intimidated by this assignment but the new me was ready. I walked into the site full of strangers and introduced myself with confidence. I communicated well in the interviews. I was at the top of my game and so were the applicants.

After interviewing candidates for a couple of days, I started to realize that something great was about to happen there. The pool of applicants was outstanding – great experience and talent. This was going to be the sales center to beat. If I could get in on the ground floor here and prove myself, I would have a shot at a mid-level position within a year. That was my plan; God had something better in mind.

It was an interesting twist of fate. We were all in a meeting to debrief the interviews. Out of nowhere a question came up about the make-up of the new site. The regional sales executive shared that the center was slated to open in March, occupy two floors, and eventually grow to 200 people. Then he said it – there would be one mid-level leadership position. My ears perked up. I began to smile. I was at the right place at the right time. This was my chance and I was going to take it.

Immediately upon returning to Virginia, I went to my manager – the same one that turned me down for promotions twice -- and expressed an interest in the leadership position in Charlotte. I could tell he was caught off guard. This was a bold move. Was I really willing to leave everything I knew? Was I truly ready to step out on faith? It was a fair question. I had spent my entire life – 34 years – in Virginia. My whole family lived there. I knew no one in Charlotte. I would be nearly 300 miles from home. It would mean starting over from ground zero. He wondered if I had the guts to go through with it. "If I tell him (the regional executive) you're interested, this is going to go really fast. Are you sure?" I didn't bat an eye. "Yes, I'm sure." In a matter of days, I was contacted for an interview and shortly thereafter I was offered the job. Without hesitation I accepted and in two weeks, I packed up and moved to Charlotte. It was one of the best decisions I have ever made – and the boldest.

Looking back, it's still somewhat hard to believe that I took that step, but I am glad I did. I now consider Charlotte home. I have a close network of friends that feel like family. I couldn't imagine living anywhere else. And it all started with walking into that room full of strangers that day. It started with believing that I was worthy; that I had something to offer the world; that I was important. For so many years I didn't believe that. Now I do.

<u>I Believe</u>

You may think it is an exaggeration to state that losing over 100 pounds changed everything, but it's true. I literally became a new person, the person I believe I was always meant to be. It wasn't just about the physical weight that I shed; it was the psychological and emotional weight as well. I no longer had to hide behind the guilt and the shame of "I could've," "I would've" or "I should've." I had taken charge of my life. Sure, some things were still out of my control, but I was doing what I could and letting God handle the rest. I was no longer allowing my emotions and insecurities to rule me. My mindset was changing. I was a believer – not just in God or in other people – but I was a believer in me.

Oh and in case you're wondering, I did re-enter the dating scene, this time with a renewed confidence. When I smell BS, I run. When men don't recognize my worth and try to take advantage of me, I tell them to take a hike. And when I sense that I'm being treated like a sex object, I let them know – I am more than that, much more than that. I will not be objectified. I will not be minimized. I will not be discounted. I am a woman, a strong, independent woman, and I will be treated as such. That's not to say I don't need a man; I'm not on that bandwagon. I want to get married; I want to have kids, but not at any cost. My dignity and self-respect must remain intact. I've fought too hard to get here and I will not go back.

Self-esteem is a tricky subject. It's based on what you think about you, which may be shaped by the opinions you believe others have about you. Thought patterns are not easy to change. It can take months, even years to make a dent depending on the person and how much emotional damage has been done. The truth is I am still working through old self-esteem issues. I sometimes find myself mentally stuck between the person I was and the person I am becoming. What has helped me bridge the gap is working on my self-respect. For me, having self-respect led to me thinking better of myself and thinking better of myself led to higher self-esteem. As my self-esteem improved, I became more confident. As my confidence grew, I began to experience breakthrough. You can experience the same.

## 3 WAYS TO BOOST YOUR SELF-CONFIDENCE

1. **Expose your mind to truth.** Many of the thoughts that plague our minds are our own. Some are based in reality and some are not. It's time to cut through the noise.

   Here are four for you to digest and meditate on:

   A. _Your size is not your worth._ A person that weighs 150 pounds is not more valuable than a person that weighs 400 pounds. Size measures how big something or someone is, in relation to something else. It does not determine your worth. Your quality of life will instantly improve when you stop believing that what size you wear makes you less valuable.

   B. _Attractiveness is subjective._ They say beauty is in the eye of the beholder which implies that beauty is relative. What one person finds attractive may not be attractive to another. For this reason, you cannot rely on what other people think; it's what you think that counts. You are the only person that is able to truly determine how worthy you are, how sexy you are, how attractive you are, how you feel about your body. People are entitled to their opinions, but those opinions cannot and should not be your driving force. They don't get to decide your worth or what is or is not appropriate for you. That's for you to decide. Only you.

   C. _Beauty and health are independent topics._ I believe the "big, beautiful woman" movement has noble intentions – improving the self-esteem and body image of the overweight. Having personally experienced the prejudice associated with being obese, I support the self-love aspect of the message. No one should feel down on themselves or less worthy of love because of their size. I believe, however, that we should love ourselves enough to live.

Self-love isn't just about you feeling good about yourself; it's about you doing what's good for you in the long-term. It's self-care. You have to take care of you too. Let's not lose sight of the facts. The statistics don't lie – four out of five African American women are overweight or obese. The evidence is clear—poor eating habits and a lack of physical activity are common among the overweight and obese. The outlook is dim – obesity and its associated behaviors increase our risk for disease and premature death.

I say it's time for some tough love. Yes, you can be big and beautiful, but when you're dead, beauty doesn't matter. Dead and beautiful is still dead. If you want to live and enjoy you're your life, you've got to invest the time and energy now. If you don't, it's a gamble. Maybe you'll squeak by without enduring disease or facing early death. Maybe you won't! Do you really want to leave your life and the quality of it to chance?

D. *People are selfish.* Yes, I said it. People are selfish. As you start to face these truths and begin taking action, not everyone will be supportive. There are cultural and individual biases that contradict with what you now know is right for you. When friends and family members tell you that you are "getting too skinny" when you know you have more weight to lose or the men in your life encourage you to stop losing weight if certain body parts start to get smaller, you need to ask yourself what is driving that. Are they looking out for their best interest or yours? Understand that as you change, it changes the way others feel about you. It also changes the way others feel about themselves. Insecurity often surfaces. He may fear losing the new you to another man. Your sister may fear that you will now get all of the attention instead of her. Your girlfriend, who is also overweight, may now feel unsettled because you are taking action and she is not.

155

Don't underestimate what people will do to retain control. Let them know you love them but remember that you are the only person that gets to decide what is appropriate for you. No one else. Self-love is also standing up for yourself and what you know is right.

2. ***Act your way into feeling.*** You act your way into feeling, not the other way around. If you're waiting to feel motivated to eat healthily and/or exercise regularly, you could be waiting a long time. Feelings are fickle. They can't be trusted. One minute you feel like doing one thing and the next minute you feel like doing completely different. Because our feelings are all over the place, they should be viewed as *indicators* and not the determinants of what we will or will not do.

Feelings don't consider long-term consequences, only the right here and right now. The truth is that in the long term you will feel better if you take control of your health, eat more nutritious foods, and become physically active. Sure, it will be rough at first. It's called an adjustment period. Yes, your mind, body, and soul will need time to adjust to your new lifestyle. It won't change overnight. It also won't change unless you start and keep at it.

Once your total self realizes that this is for real, it will adjust and you will love the benefits of your new life – more energy, greater mental focus, a vibrant appearance. You just have to get over the hump. Be patient. Give yourself time to get there. You will get there.

3. ***Do it Daily.*** Daily decisions determine destiny – emotionally, mentally, and physically. Good self-esteem doesn't just happen. It isn't just a matter of you saying nice things about and to yourself.

Without any other change in behavior, habits, and environment, you will not automatically stop thinking bad things about yourself and start thinking good things. If you make poor eating choices and don't exercise on a daily basis, *things aren't going to get better and you shouldn't expect them to.* It doesn't happen by osmosis. Yes, God will help you but you need to do your part. It takes intentionality. It takes effort. It may even take sweat and tears, but it can be done. It has to be done daily. One day a week of healthy eating will not erase six days poor eating. It just doesn't work that day.

And remember, you can't rely on feeling like doing it every day. Five years later, I still don't feel like doing it every day. What gets me out of the bed in the morning and into my home gym is remembering this: the decisions you make today will determine your tomorrow. We often forget that decisions add up over time through the miracle of compounding. What seems small and insignificant today, when done repeatedly, produces major and woefully significant consequences later. High blood pressure, diabetes, heart disease and cancer don't just appear out of the blue. They are the result of years of poor daily decisions.

The good news is you can decide differently, starting today. The even better news is that if you start today and keep at it, you can reverse the effects of previous poor decisions. I am a witness -- you can reclaim your life. Starting today.

Reflection Points:

1. Which of the four truths hits home the most? How has believing the lie been holding you back?
2. How intentional have you been about taking control of your health?
3. What actions can you take to improve your tomorrow starting today?

# Chapter 20 - Gutsy Girl Emerges

Living life without limits…what does that mean to you? To me, it means being able to look at a gigantic task that is before me and think "I can" instead of "I can't." We all face giants. Some are mental and emotional. Others are physical. There is often an undertone of fear. "Will I look like a fool?" "What will so-and-so think?" We weigh ourselves down with this psychological baggage and wonder why we aren't living up to our full potential. Well at least I did. Maybe you can identify.

<u>Life without Limits</u>

After a day of team building activities with my fellow MBA cohorts, I realized how I had limited myself. There were all kinds of fun and exciting things that I wasn't doing because 1) I wasn't exposed to them, 2) was out of shape and 3) I feared embarrassment. I had put myself in a box. Get up, go to work, come home, watch TV, go to sleep and repeat. That was my every day existence. On weekends, I hung out with family and friends at their home or mine, went out to eat, did a little shopping, but that was about it. The last time I had done anything remotely similar to an obstacle course was in high school. I had never rock climbed in my life. A tight rope exercise? Please. That was not on my list of exciting things to do…until that fateful day in January.

> *"I'm about to lose control and I think I like it!"*
> *~"I'm So Excited," The Pointer Sisters*

Although I was horrified and terribly embarrassed that day, I learned something about myself. I liked thrill and adventure! Now maybe I should have had a clue because I had always had a passion for rollercoasters. Even though the trek to the top scared me, I loved the thrill of coming down the hill at top speed then sweeping up again. The twists and the turns, exciting! I got a rush every time! The obstacle course, rock climbing and tight rope exercise gave me that same type of rush. Maybe it was the air of predictability that I loved; allowing myself to lose control and not know the outcome in advance was exhilarating! Pushing myself to go beyond what I thought capable was challenging and amazing at the same time. There was something wonderful about pushing through the fear and coming out victorious. I loved that feeling and I wanted desperately to repeat it - minus being out of shape and consequently being embarrassed by my performance, of course. And I would.

Today some of my favorite activities are zip lining, white water rafting, and jet skiing. Parasailing, sky diving and scuba diving remain on my bucket list. These are all activities that would have scared the living day lights out of me before. I wouldn't dare think about doing them. But today, I am strong in my conviction that I have the ability to conquer, or at least, complete outdoor physical activities. That assurance didn't come out of thin air. It came from overcoming challenges I once thought to be impossible at home - in my home gym to be exact.

*Hip Hop Abs* will always be my first love but my journey in fitness didn't stop there. I have over 25 different workout programs in my home gym and I'm constantly adding more. Every 60-90 days I give myself a new challenge to keep from getting bored, ensure I continue to get results, and test my perceived limits. I started out just wanting to be healthy and gained a passion for fitness. Maybe you will too.

## It Pays to Be Fit

There are a lot of misconceptions about fitness. It is not a svelte body or a "cut" appearance. Those things are sometimes byproducts but not always. Our level of fitness is a measure of our ability to perform physical activity. It is generally achieved through proper nutrition, exercise, hygiene and rest, but let me be clear, you can be fit and fat. I wasn't, but it is possible. I'm going make another controversial statement: It's better to be fat and fit than skinny and unfit.

In a 2007 death rates study published in The Journal of the American Medical Association and later covered by the NY Times,[27] there was a striking revelation -- death rates among the overweight, those with a B.M.I. of 25 to 30, were slightly lower than in normal weight adults. As a side note, death rates were highest among those with a B.M.I. of 35 or more. The study brought to light that fitness level is the strongest predictor of mortality risk regardless of B.M.I. Participants who exhibited a lower level of fitness, as measured on treadmill tests, were four times more likely to die during the 12-year study than those with the highest level of fitness. And get this: Participants with a minimal level of fitness were 50% less likely to die an early death when compared with those who were least fit (and in some instances skinny). In case you're wondering, the results were adjusted to control for age, smoking and underlying heart problems. Even after all of those adjustments, fitness, not weight, was the most prevalent factor in forecasting death rates. The moral of the story? It's not just about fatness; fitness matters...for everyone.

## A Culture in Crisis

Being fat in and of itself is not the problem. It's the lifestyle that is typically associated with an overweight or obese person – fast food and junk food, the absence of portion control, and little-to-no physical activities. There is a strong correlation between these behaviors and the likelihood that a person will be overweight and therefore at greater risk for disease. That doesn't mean, however, that an overweight person can't be healthy. It is less likely, but not impossible. If that person eats right more often than not, is physically active, and gets the proper rest, they can (and most likely are) healthy. Unfortunately, such a lifestyle is not the norm for the average overweight person. In fact it is quite the opposite, especially for African Americans.

*Fast Facts:*

- In 2011, African Americans were 1.5 times as likely to be obese as Non-Hispanic Whites.[28]
- In 2010, African Americans were 70% less likely to engage in active physical activity as Non-Hispanic Whites.[29]
- African Americans consume less than 1 serving of whole grains per day.[30]
- 7% of African Americans consume 2 or more cups of fruit per day.[31]
- 3% of African Americans consume 2.5 or more cups of vegetables per day.[32]
- African American men consume an average of 3.6 servings of processed meats per week.[33]
- 65% of African Americans consume 5 or more servings of sugar-sweetened beverages per week.[34]
- 66%of African Americans consume 2.5 servings or more of sweets and bakery desserts per week.[35]

*This is despite the fact that:*

- Nearly 60% of obese African American adults were given advice about exercise.[36]
- 50% of those who were obese were given advice about eating fewer high fat or high cholesterol foods.[37]

What do I want you to take away from all of this? Focus on doing the right things and the right results will follow. The desired result will be different for every individual. For some that will include getting to a certain weight. For others it will be simply achieving a specific level of fitness. You get to define what success looks like for you. You don't, however, get to change the facts. The facts are that everyone that wants a good quality of life - one free of sickness and disease; a life without limits, needs to eat balanced meals, be active, and get 7-8 hours of sleep per day, regardless of size. Those are the facts.

You may even find, as I have, that there is an adventurer buried deep inside that has been waiting to get out. You may find that as your level of fitness improves, you become more willing to try new things. You become more open. More free.

Like the wondrous caterpillar that morphs into a butterfly, after a few months in your cocoon of healthy living your body radically transforms. You emerge stronger. You have less fear. You are a champion. Nothing can stand in your way. That's what a life without limits is all about. Want in?

> *"If you always put limits on everything you do, physical or anything else. It will spread into your work and into your life. There are no limits. There are only plateaus, and you must not stay there, you must go beyond them."*
> ~Bruce Lee

## 5 STEPS TO FIND YOUR INNER ADVENTURER

1. **Find a workout you love.** In the beginning I don't want you to focus on finding the workout that burns the most calories, makes you the sorest, or kicks your butt the most. I want you to find something that you actually somewhat enjoy and look forward to doing (once you get past the normal pre-exercise blahs). I want you to not hate it. The chances of you sticking with something you hate, especially in the beginning are slim to none. It may take you trying a variety of things – home workout DVDs, fitness classes at the gym, a couch to 5K program, sports, or weight lifting routine – to figure out what works for you. Right now, your mission is simply to find a workout you like enough to continue.

2. **Start small.** You can reverse the effects of years' worth of poor decisions, but it isn't done overnight. Set yourself up for success by starting small – as little as 10 minutes a day – until you get the

hang of that and then build from there. You don't need to lift the heaviest weight in the gym or go the hardest in your class. You don't even need to keep up with the participants in your class, live or on DVD. The only person you are competing with is you. Are you giving it your personal best? Are you testing your limits? If the answers to those questions are yes, you are a success. Any voice that says otherwise is lying to you. Don't burn yourself out with unrealistic expectations. You will eventually get to 20 minutes, 30 minutes or more. Give yourself time to get there.

3. **Switch it up.** They say that variety is the spice of life; this is true for fitness as well. I loved *Hip Hop Abs* in the beginning and still do today. But if I did that workout every day for the last 5 years, I would be bored to tears! I also would have ceased to get results. You have to constantly think out of the box and mix it up. This is something you are doing for life, not just for 90 days or a year. In order for this to be a lifetime process vs. a one-time event, you have to explore different types of workouts; you have to try new things. Don't wait until you reach a certain size to start living; keep challenging what you think is possible for you. You are stronger than you think!

4. **Have a plan.** I've said it before and I'll say it again. What doesn't get planned doesn't get done. We are all full of good intentions, but good health isn't the product of intentions. It is the result of consistent, positive action. In order to be consistent you've got to create an exercise plan each week. Your life isn't the same every week; your exercise plan shouldn't be either. Some days you will need to work out at 5:00 AM. Others you can do 6:00 AM. Some weeks you will have to do evenings. You need to have a DVD at home for when your schedule doesn't allow for the drive to the gym. Plan the days and times you will work out in advance. Put it on your smartphone calendar or print out a paper version, whatever works for you.

5. **Remember Why You Are Doing It.** This is not just about wearing a certain size, looking good for your best friend's wedding or your upcoming vacation. This is about your quality of

life, now and in the future. It's about living to a ripe old age and enjoying all that retirement has to offer. It's about increasing your stamina and ability to perform at work, in the community and at home. It's about living to see your grandkids. It's about fulfilling your God-given purpose. It's about living your best life. That's what you really want, right?

## Reflection Points

1. How many servings of fruits and vegetables do you eat per day? Is that okay? (Hint: The recommendation is five to nine servings per day)
2. How would scheduling your workouts in advance help you? What challenges could you face and how could you deal with them?

26. Psychologytoday.com, 2008

27. NY Times, 2008

28. Minorityhealth.hhs.gov, 2013

29. Minorityhealth.hhs.gov, 2013

30 - 35. Heart.org, 2013

36 – 37. Minorityhealth.hhs.gov, 2013

# Chapter 21 – Addicted to Energy

I spent at least 8 years of my life addicted to food. I now consider myself a recovering "foodaholic." I still love food. I love the look of it, the taste of it, the texture of it, and the smell of it. I've grown to have an appreciation for and love of nutritious food, but I'd be lying if I told you my taste for the not-so-healthy stuff just disappeared. As a matter-of-fact, as I type, I am resisting the temptation to cut myself a hefty slice of 6 layer chocolate cake leftover from our Thanksgiving festivities. I am still a work in progress. I hope I make it (smile).

<u>Another Vice</u>

I am happy to say, though, that I'm now addicted to the benefits of my new life. One of the primary ones being energy. Energy is defined as "the strength and vitality required for sustained physical or mental activity." Strength and vitality were not a part of my former life. As a matter-of-fact, even when I was younger and thinner, I wasn't this alive. I didn't feel *this* good. I wasn't this strong – mentally, emotionally, or physically. Health and fitness changed me and changed me for good.

Many people are aware of how a healthy lifestyle benefits them physically. Let's talk about the mental and emotional aspects of physical fitness.

## *PHYSICAL FITNESS…*

1. ***Requires concentration.*** Concentration is the ability to stay focused on and be fully aware of what is going on around you. For example, in performing the moves in my home workout DVDs, I have to pay close attention to what is being demonstrated – the pace, the rhythm, the intensity, the form, in order to duplicate it. I have to be my own coach, correcting my mistakes and patting myself on the back for getting it right. I can't afford to get distracted. If I do, the best case is I won't get the best results; worst case is that I'll suffer an injury. Neither is an outcome that compliments my goals.

2. ***Builds discipline.*** Being able to convince yourself to go to the gym when you'd rather head home and lay on the couch requires discipline. Choosing fruits and veggies over fries requires will power. Deciding to eat within 30 to 60 minutes of finishing your workout requires planning – and discipline. A fit lifestyle isn't easy. It's work. That's why many quit even though they desire a better life.

   A person who has committed to fitness, on the other hand, has somehow managed to focus more on the long-term benefits than the short-term sacrifices. They've zeroed in on what's most important and have designed their life in a way that aligns with their goals.

3. ***Produces persistence.*** That moment when you want to quit and you find the strength to go for one more minute or do one more rep, you could easily say, "I'm exhausted" or "it's too heavy" but you don't. After a while, you learn that the voice in your head is a liar. You figure out that your mind will almost always quit on you before you reach your physical limit. You are capable of much, much more than you think. But without a history of proving that this is true, you give up, even when the finish line is in sight.

   Fitness teaches you the value of persistence – of staying the course. It reminds you that you will win; you will cross the line…if you don't quit.

4. **Strengthens mental toughness.** This may sound contradictory but fitness is 90% mental and about 10% physical. What I mean by that is that you can be out of shape and outperform a physically fit person if you are stronger in mindset. Just think about it, people have been known to do amazing things when the pressure is on. An overweight woman will literally run into a burning building at top speed to save her daughter. An obese man will lift a car off the ground to free his son who is trapped underneath. Given the right incentive, we are capable of just about anything. Being fit certainly makes these tasks easier but mental toughness is what really separates people that fail from people that succeed.

When you accomplish things you previously thought you could not do, you start to think differently. You see yourself in a different light. You become unstoppable; not just in dire circumstances but every day. You become an everyday hero.

I struggled in all of these areas prior to developing a fit lifestyle. I lost focus easily, especially when doing tasks I didn't particularly care for. I catered to my feelings more than I should have. Not just in terms of eating and exercise, but in relationships and in my career. I often took the easy way out. I didn't have the mindset of a finisher. But the more fit and persistent I became -- the more I was able to handle the tough stuff. I didn't have to be assured that I would win before I would begin. I came to realize that success was more than winning. Sometimes success is being willing to attempt; being open to the possibility of failure. It's realizing that pain is temporary but quitting on myself, has consequences that endure time and space.

> *"Pain is temporary. It may last for a minute, or an hour or a day, or even a year. But eventually, it will subside. And something else takes its place. If I quit, however, it will last forever."*
> *~Lance Armstrong*

Just in case you are unfamiliar, let's talk briefly about the physical energy that fitness creates. Physical benefits include improved:

- Endurance
- Strength
- Coordination
- Balance
- Posture
- Agility
- Cognitive (brain) function
- Sleep

It's important to consider that fitness isn't just about being able to "go hard" in the gym, run a marathon, or compete in a *Tough Mudder*. It's also about preparing the body for every day, real-world activities. It's about having a better quality of life. Wouldn't it be nice to be able to perform daily activities without pain or being winded? Things like:

- Lifting your kids
- Carrying groceries
- Climbing the stairs
- Bending down to pick up something that fell
- Reaching for items on the top shelf
- Enjoying play time with your children
- Catching yourself and avoiding injury during a fall

This isn't an exhaustive list, but it gives you an idea of how your life can be different if you make fitness a priority.

This is your chance. You don't have to remain fatigued and lethargic. You have a large degree of control over how you feel. Get moving and watch your mental, emotional, and physical energy rise.

I love the way the fit life feels. You will too.

## 4 WAYS TO MAXIMIZE THE ENERGY YOU RECEIVE FROM EXERCISE

1. **Fuel up and fuel properly.** While some contend that you should workout out on an empty stomach, it is important that you have

enough energy to fuel your workout. If your stomach is growling the whole time and all you can think about is food, you're highly unlikely to give the workout your best. When you don't give the workout your best, you hamper your results.

Remember that food is energy. Keep your stomach happy by enjoying a small protein and carbohydrate snack (ex. Banana or 1 small slice of whole wheat bread for carbs and 1-2 tablespoons of natural peanut butter or a small cup of yogurt for protein) 30-45 minutes before you exercise. Or eat a healthy meal on your regular schedule and wait 1.5-2 hours before your exercise.

2. ***Reduce stress and get your rest.*** Fitness guru Tony Horton says this about the connection between stress, sleep and fitness: "Stressed out, sleep-deprived people don't eat right and exercise regularly. Stress depletes energy, strength, and desire; poor sleep habits affect your moods and immune function along with cognitive and motor performance. Burning the candle at both ends makes it impossible to be fit and healthy." Let us aim to get 7-8 hours of quality sleep per night.

As a side note, you may want to avoid rigorous activity 3-4 hours before bed. Body temperature rises when you exercise, which may make it harder for you to get to sleep (happens to me every time!).

3. ***Soak in some sun.*** Several scientific studies suggest that sunlight positively influences mood and alertness. For this reason, you may want to consider an outdoor workout or carving out a few minutes a day to relax in the sunshine on your deck. I think that you will come to the same conclusion that researchers have - sunshine helps to brighten your outlook on life.

4. ***Build a playlist of high-energy tunes.*** I hate to break it to you, but here is the cold, hard truth: there will be days when you won't even feel like doing your "soul mate" workout. Working out can be mind-numbing at times. You won't always feel motivated.

One way to find the fortitude to power though is to fire up your favorite tunes. Like sunshine, I find music to be an almost instant mood lifter. Try it. I bet it will work for you too.

Reflection Points

1. How could living a fit lifestyle help you have a better quality of life?
2. How many hours of sleep do you typically get per night? Is that okay?

# Chapter 22 – Mind Relief

My doctor really rocked my world with the "you're going to be sick or worse" thing. Five years later, those words still echo in my mind. I didn't like the idea of being sick, but "or worse"? I didn't even know how to process that. The thought that someone – me in particular – could actually *die* as a result of what boiled down to repeated poor decision-making; that some forms of disease were self-inflicted, I hadn't fully considered that. It was a weighty thought. Like a drug addict, I had been chasing "the high" not realizing that one day the chase would eventually kill me.

<u>Chasing Peace</u>

It has been said that "ignorance is bliss." This was certainly true for me. I had been skipping along thinking everything was okay. I felt fine and I assumed that meant I was fine, for the most part anyway. Sure, I had a few aches and pains here and there but it was nothing serious, or so I thought. After the tough love talk, my mind was completely unsettled. Thoughts of what my life could be like if I didn't change plagued my mind. I was no longer ignorant of the consequences of my decisions and those consequences became my "why."

My why became the driving force of my transformation. When I didn't feel like working out, I thought about why it was important that I did. When I was stressed and wanted to eat everything in sight, I thought about why that wasn't a good idea. Thinking about what was at stake *before* I made a decision was a game changer. I had been living much of my life on auto-pilot. I gave very little thought to the after-effects. It was all about the here and now. But with this newfound conviction, I programmed myself to think beyond the immediate. I trained myself to think about what was good for me long-term. I constantly reminded myself that daily decisions determine destiny. It all paid off.

When I reached a healthy weight in October of 2008, a huge weight was lifted off of my shoulders. For the first time in years, my blood pressure numbers were normal and I didn't have to worry about the threat of medication. There were no guarantees that my life would be disease free (there are a number of other factors in play such as race and family history), but I did have the assurance that I had done what I could. I had done my part. I had controlled what I could control. No "I wish", "I should have" or "I could have". There would be no regrets. It was such a great feeling and one that I strive to maintain. It isn't easy, but it is worth it.

Sleepwalking

I won't sugar coat it. Change is hard. If it were easy, everyone would do it. It's not and that's why many don't. If it were as simple as making good choices for 30, 60, or 90 days, we could handle that, but making good decisions for life? That will take some work, a lot of work. It will take sacrifice, a lot of sacrifice. It will take discipline, a lot of discipline. Work, sacrifice and discipline are not pleasant in the moment, but the payoff down the road is amazing. Are you willing to trade short-term pleasure for long-term gain?

Acting with purpose yields peace. Pop culture and media messages have deceived us into thinking that a carefree lifestyle - one where we don't think but feel - is the one that leads to happiness. But tell me, how often have you made a thoughtless, purely emotional decision and come out ahead? More often than not, when we allow our feelings to rule and act without consciously thinking, we get ourselves into trouble...big trouble. We say things we shouldn't say and cause animosity and strain in our most important relationships. We play when we should be working, miss deadlines or find ourselves unprepared when opportunities arise jeopardizing our futures. We watch hours of mindless TV or play around on social media when we could be praying, meditating or reading a thought-provoking (not trashy) book. And, we binge on junk food after days of being "good" and cancel out all of the hard work we've done. We didn't intend for any of these things to happen, but they do because as Darren Hardy, author of The Compound Effect, says we're sleepwalking through our choices.

> *"Your biggest challenge isn't that you've intentionally been making bad choices. Heck that would be easy to fix. Your biggest challenge is that you've been sleepwalking through your choices. Half the time, you're not even aware you're making them! Our choices are often shaped by our culture and upbringing. They can be so entwined in our routine behaviors and habits that they seem beyond our control. For instance, have you ever been going about your business, enjoying your life, when all of sudden you made a stupid choice or series of small choices that ultimately sabotaged your hard work and momentum, all for no apparent reason? You didn't intend to sabotage yourself, but by not thinking about your decisions— weighing the risks and potential outcomes—you found yourself facing unintended consequences. Nobody intends to become obese, go through bankruptcy, or get a divorce, but often (if not always) those consequences are the result of a series of small, poor choices."*
> *~Darren Hardy*

Being conscious of your choices doesn't guarantee that you will always make the "best choice." It simply means that you make thoughtful decisions. A couple of times a week, I purposely choose to give myself a mental and emotional break by deviating from a super healthy diet and enjoying a *reasonable, calculated* indulgence. The key words here, however, are reasonable and calculated. Where I used to go wrong was in indulging without a clear plan, not having a reasonableness check, and failing to exercise portion control. For example, I would kill myself in the gym and then order a Quarter Pounder with Cheese meal because 1) I didn't plan for the fact that I would be hungry after leaving the gym, 2) I had no concept of how many calories I had just burned with exercise or how many I was about to eat, 3) I wrongly assumed that what was served to me was a sensible portion. I made a conscious choice to go the gym because it was the right thing to do, but I slept through the rest of it! How often are you halfway thinking through your choices?

The truth is no matter how good we claim to be, we all sleep walk at times. It's a part of being human. We easily form habits, short cuts if you will, that make life easier because we just go with the flow and don't have to think. It's one of our greatest weaknesses because bad habits are hard to break. The good news is we can choose to act differently. When we act differently, we plant the seeds for new habits. If we cultivate them, they will grow and eventually overpower our bad habits, most of the time. Perfection is allusive, but excellence is achievable. If I can do it, you can do it too.

## 7 TIPS TO RECLAIM YOUR PEACE AND YOUR HEALTH

1. ***Stop Saying Yes.*** No doubt you've heard the exhortation to "just say no" before. First Lady Nancy Reagan created and made this saying popular in the 80's to discourage children from saying yes to recreational drugs, violence and premarital sex. I say it's time that adults started taking heed and that we expand the list to include self-destructive behaviors that we don't talk about as much: approval addiction, emotional eating, overeating, inactivity, and overcommitting.

   If we're going to change for the better, we have to stop saying yes to people's requests because we are afraid of how they will react if we say no. We have to stop saying yes to the brownies, cupcakes, and ice cream when we're all out of indulgences for the week. We have to learn to stop saying yes to the voice that says, "Just one more bite," when we are already full. We have to stop saying yes to the couch, lace up our shoes and head to the gym because we said we would. We must check our calendar, interest and energy level before committing to another engagement no matter how awesome the cause.

To change your life and reclaim your peace, you must learn to say no. It doesn't mean that you don't do things to please yourself or others, but rather that you do it how and when it's appropriate. No more mindless decision making.

2. ***Figure Out What YOU Really Want.*** One of the biggest ah ha's I've had on my journey is that our choices are largely influenced by our environment. Translation: Many of the things you say, do, and believe today are the result of cultural norms and your upbringing and have nothing to do with what you *really* believe and want.

For example, in some African American communities being "big-boned," or "thick," is to be desired and those that are thinner are given disparaging labels like "stick and bones." As a result, some African American women prioritize having a certain look above reaching a healthy weight. But where did this all come from? Is the "thick" look what these ladies really want or is it simply what they've been conditioned to believe is appropriate? Just as the "big-boned" and "thick" ideologies drive the decisions of some African American women, many of the decisions you make today are not even your own.

My challenge to you: instead of always doing what you've always done, it's time that you begin questioning *why* you are doing what you're doing. Ask yourself questions like:

- Why do I always do X when Y happens?
- Where did I learn this?
- Is this what *I* really want? Or what someone else wants for me?
- Will the decision I am about to make bring me closer to my goal or take me further away?

175

- Am I making this decision to please others or because it aligns with my goals or makes me happy?

It's ultra-important that you don't allow cultural norms and learned behaviors to rule simply because you didn't take the time to vote.

3. ***Keep it Real.*** Making a lifestyle change can be difficult. Make it easier on yourself by explaining to your family and friends what you plan to accomplish, why it is important to you, and how it will benefit them. For example, explain that losing 30 pounds will bring your blood pressure/cholesterol/blood sugar levels in line and improve your overall health. Also, don't be afraid to share how the excess weight is affecting your quality of life as well as theirs. It may be helpful to explain that at your current weight you haven't been feeling well, have less energy, etc. Then share how losing it will allow you to spend more quality time with *them* doing the things they love. A similar approach can be used with your friends. The people that truly love you will want you to look and feel your best.

4. ***Speak Up and Be Specific.*** In most instances, our family and friends want us to be successful, but they don't always know how to help us succeed. Remove the guesswork by getting specific about how they can help you. If you need your spouse or one of your older children to watch the baby for 45 minutes, 3 times a week to free up some time for your workouts, say so. If you need accountability, share the specifics of your eating plan and ask your family to help you stick to it by not bringing junk food in the house, keeping it in an area that you don't frequent, or at the very least not eating it in front of you. If your girlfriends have a tendency to tempt you by offering you a "treat," ask them to stop. Their intentions are innocent – wanting to relieve you of some of the stress that's involved in making a lifestyle change – but they may not realize that their actions are hurting rather than helping. Or maybe they do and they are a saboteur. In any event, make it clear what you need.

5. ***Bring in the Reinforcements.*** If you have kept it real and been specific about the support you need but your friends and family still aren't supportive, I would suggest you re-evaluate those relationships. I'm not saying disown them, but I am suggesting that you limit your interactions and find your support elsewhere.

Research shows that having the proper support greatly improves your chances of success. Pair up with someone at the gym, on the job, at church, or in your neighborhood that has similar goals or has been there and can coach you through it. You may also find success by joining a weight loss program or fitness support group. If you need that one-on-one personal touch, perhaps hiring a personal trainer, nutritionist, dietician, or fitness coach will do the trick. The bottom line is surrounding yourself with positive approaches to weight loss (and people you can share your challenges and victories with), will make your journey much easier.

6. ***De-stress, De-clutter and Re-organize.*** Have you ever noticed how coming home to a messy home dampens your spirits? Or how walking into a disorganized office makes you feel overwhelmed? Believe it or not, your home and work environment will play a big role in determining whether or not you reach your goals. You'll need to minimize stress in these areas to offset the added stress of making a lifestyle change.

First, create a "no stress zone" at home. This can be as simple as a comfortable chair and a lamp nestled in the corner of your bedroom to provide an escape. Second, clean out your kitchen. Get rid of foods that will derail you or at the very least take them out of plain sight. Ensure that foods that promote your new lifestyle are readily available and easily accessible. Enjoy the occasional indulgence outside of the home so that you aren't tempted to overdo it. Third, establish a sense of order at work. Create a to-do list at the end of the day so that you know where to start the next day. Clean off your desk or at least stack the papers nicely so that you aren't overwhelmed when you walk in the door. Come up with a system for managing daily tasks (emails, reviewing reports, preparing presentations, etc.) so there is always a degree of control (even if everything else is outside of your control). By creating a healthy home and work environment, you are setting yourself up to be more motivated and committed to reaching your weight loss goals. Don't let these things rob you of your peace for one more day.

7. ***Take it One Day at a Time.*** I've said it before and I'll say it again, change takes time. Don't burn yourself out by demanding too much too soon. Take it one step and one day at a time. Rather than trying to give your life a complete overhaul all at once, try implementing one change – eating habits or exercise – at a time. Or make small changes in both areas. You know what you can realistically handle without sending yourself over the edge. Past experience has taught you that.

One of the ways you can show yourself love is to be patient. The Good Book teaches that the race is not given to the swift or to the strong, but to the one that endures. Your goal is to finish, not be the first person to cross the finish line.

Reflection Points

1. In what areas have you been sleepwalking through your choices?
2. What do you need to stop saying yes to?
3. What do YOU really want?

> *"If you don't design your own life plan, chances are you'll fall into someone else's plan. And guess what they have planned for you? Not much."*
> *~Jim Rohn*

# Realistic Journey

With the powerful combination of patience, persistence, and prayer, I have lost a total of 110 lbs. and over 10 inches in my waist. I now wear a size 6/8. I've appeared on Dr. Oz with my fitness coach Shaun T. and my success is currently being featured in a top-selling infomercial. As proud as I am of those accomplishments, I'm more proud of the person I've become.

I've learned to love myself. I am teaching myself to strive for excellence rather than perfection. I've learned how to enjoy life without going overboard. I've gained a passion for fitness and pushing my limits. I've developed an appreciation and love for healthy foods. I've taught myself that it is okay to be consistently imperfect. I now live life without limits.

I hope by sharing my story that you can see that I'm no extraordinary person. I have had the same battles and challenges as everyone else. The only difference is that I found the courage to change, came up with a realistic plan, and stuck with it. During my transformation I had good days and bad days – and still do, but hear this: I refuse to quit! No matter how many times I fall off the wagon – yes, I still do – I will not go back. I have too much to lose – renewed confidence, good health and peace of mind. Absolutely priceless.

The secret to weight loss really isn't a secret. It really boils down to two things – eating healthy and staying active. Sound pretty simple? It is, but admittedly, it's not easy. Nothing worth having is. It will require grit and resilience but is *not* mission impossible. Anyone can do it and that includes you.

It IS possible. You just have to believe.

# APPENDIX
*Blank Worksheets*

# GOAL SETTING WORKSHEET

1. **Decide on a 30-day goal and why it's important.** Note: If your why isn't powerful enough to make you hit the gym when you'd rather relax or pass on your favorite dessert, it needs some work!

_____

_____

_____

_____

2. **Decide how much you are willing to "pay." What sacrifices are you willing to make <u>consistently</u> for the next 30 days?**

   a. _____

   _____

   b. _____

   _____

   c. _____

   _____

   d. _____

   _____

3. **Do a sanity check:**

   a. Does #2 align with #1? In other words, is what you are willing to pay enough to get you to your goal?

   _____

   _____

   _____

   b. Is it something you can <u>reasonably</u> accomplish in the next 30 days? Do you have some "grace" built into your plan?

_____

_____

_____

*Important: If the answer to either of these questions is* <u>*no*</u>*, go back and revise your goal!*

4. **Decide how you will reward yourself when you achieve your goal.** Make sure your reward does not conflict with your goal, meaning neither rewards or punishments should have anything to do with food or exercise. Additionally, **decide on the penalty if you do not reach it.** Attaching good and negative consequences increases your chances of success.

If I reach my goal I will:

_____

_____


If I do not reach my goal I will:

_____

_____

# BEHAVIORAL CONTRACT

Behavioral contracting is an effective behavior-modification strategy where you set up a system of rewards for sticking to the lifestyle-modification program. Behavioral contracting is most effective when the rewards are outlined by you, meaningful to you and **do not involve food or exercise**. If the rewards are not meaningful, you may not find them to be worth working toward. Behavioral contracting works differently for each individual. You are encouraged to set goals that will work for you rather than trying to duplicate others. Additionally, behavioral contracting is most effective when it is used consistently. Once you are certain the goals you outline below are met, you will set new goals.

**I Will:**

New Behavior (What):

1. _____
2. _____
3. _____

Starting (When)

1. _____
2. _____
3. _____

Frequency (How Often)

1. _____
2. _____
3. _____

This is Important to Me Because (Why)

_____

_____

How confident am I that I will do this? ___ (on a scale of 0 to 10, with 0 being not at all confident and 10 being completely confident).

If I successfully make this positive lifestyle change by _____ , I will reward myself with _____.

If I fail to successfully make this positive lifestyle change, I will forfeit this reward.

I, _____, have reviewed this contract and I agree to discuss the experience involved in accomplishing or not accomplishing this health behavior improvement with _____ (my accountability partner) on _____.

Signed:

_____

(Goal Setter)

Signed:

_____

(Witness)